As a mother of four under-5 year olds, and with a busy job, one of the most daunting things I found after having each child was to find the time to even think about getting my body back. As every mum knows, best-laid plans will often get snowballed by the family.

Fit and Fabulous for life after babies is for me, and all mums, looking for a way to balance life by incorporating a realistic, no fads, supportive and informative blueprint to achieve the ultimate goal of getting 'me' back. Fiona Thomas Hargraves provides simple, yet effective exercise techniques and food guidelines that can easily fit into an average mum's day, and there are shopping lists, too! Most importantly, this book is very big on flexibility and always having a plan B.

Fiona's approach is such a refreshing change from today's celebrity ambush of 'stick thin, post-baby body' mums as she provides us with the tools to make us feel good about ourselves in a realistic way, and tips on how to include fitness with the other 1000 things we have to juggle as mums.

After reading it I felt empowered and thought, 'Yep I can do this'. Goodbye guilt—hello body!

NICOLE SHEFFIELD
Mother of 4; General Manger, Lifestytle Channel
and Lifestyle FOOD; and *Sunrise* All-Star

'Looking after yourself is the best gift you that can give your children.' This simple statement underlines the powerful message of Fiona Thomas Hargraves' book, *Fit and Fabulous for life after babies*. The key to successful parenting is a happy and healthy mother (and father). If the parents are happy, the child will be happy. Factual but simple, this book will empower women in their reproductive years to reclaim their minds and their bodies.

DR VIJAY ROACH
Obstetrician, and Chairman, The Gidget Foundation

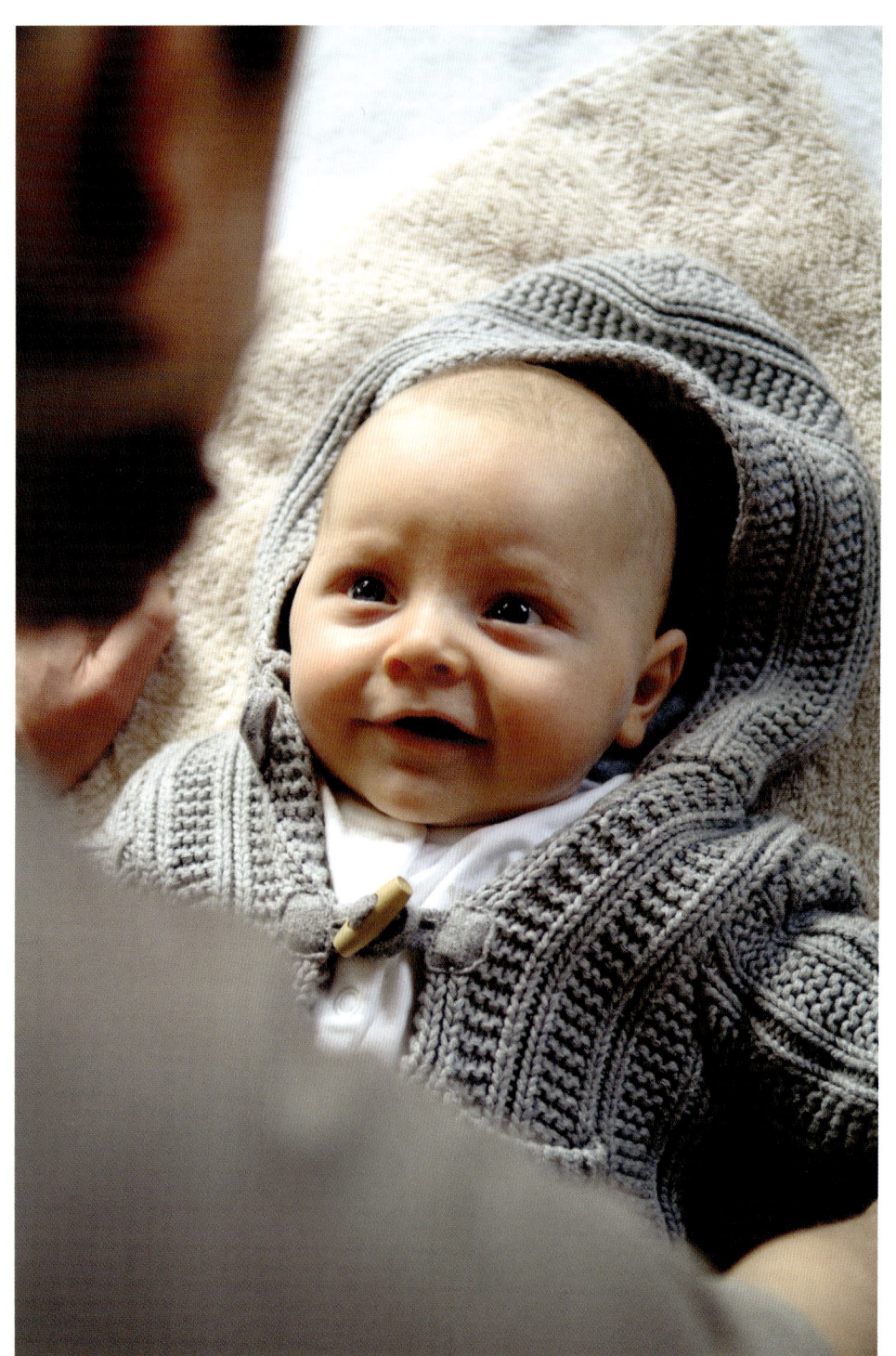

FIT & FABULOUS
FOR LIFE AFTER BABIES

FIONA THOMAS HARGRAVES

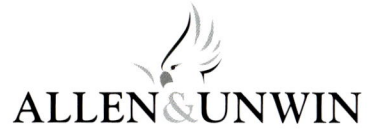

To my beautiful family without whom I wouldn't be a mother; my happy, cheeky, children, Caitlin and Lachlan and my wonderful husband Ben. You three are my inspiration.

At any stage before, during or after pregnancy, it is essential you have medical clearance before starting this program or any type of physical activity. Your doctor will be able to advise you of any precautions, considerations or modifications for your particular circumstances.

First published in 2009
Copyright © Fiona Thomas Hargraves 2009
Copyright © photographs (except front cover and page 7) Katrina Crook

All rights reserved. No part of this book may be reproduced or transmitted in any form or by any means, electronic or mechanical, including photocopying, recording or by any information storage and retrieval system, without prior permission in writing from the publisher. The *Australian Copyright Act 1968* (the Act) allows a maximum of one chapter or 10 per cent of this book, whichever is the greater, to be photocopied by any educational institution for its educational purposes provided that the educational institution (or body that administers it) has given a remuneration notice to Copyright Agency Limited (CAL) under the Act.

Allen & Unwin
83 Alexander Street
Crows Nest NSW 2065
Australia
Phone: (61 2) 8425 0100
Fax: (61 2) 9906 2218
Email: info@allenandunwin.com
Web: www.allenandunwin.com

National Library of Australia
Cataloguing-in-Publication entry:

Hargraves, Fiona Thomas.

Fit and Fabulous for life after babies / Fiona Thomas Hargraves.

978 1 74175 494 0 (pbk.)

Physical fitness for women. Mothers – Health and hygiene. Mothers – Life skills guides.

613.7045

Cover and internal design and typesetting: Liz Seymour
Set in 11/14 Fairfield Light
Printed in Singapore by KHL Printing Co Pte Ltd

10 9 8 7 6 5 4 3 2 1

Foreword

It is my pleasure to write a foreword to Fiona Thomas Hargraves' *Fit and Fabulous for life after babies*. Fiona delivers her message in a thorough, factual and authoritative style, with a gentle, unthreatening approach that is particularly valuable to women conditioned by the unachievable 'yummy mummy' construct. The clear, non-pejorative style makes this book approachable for women. Fiona's exercise regimens are detailed and comprehensive, but written with the normal woman in mind. Her dietary advice is equally thorough, but still manages to leave room for enjoyment rather than denial. Switching from the punitive 'diet', which Fiona dismisses outright, to 'eating right', she creates a positive message for women.

Fiona clearly explains the benefits to women and their babies when they combine fitness with childbearing and childrearing. She challenges the 'Supermum' myth and reassures the reader that motherhood is challenging and, indeed, sometimes overwhelming. Exercise, fitness and a healthy diet are essential to the psychological well-being of all women (and their doctors too!). The impact of appropriate lifestyle modification on mood is significant, particularly when perinatal anxiety and depression has a growing prevalence. And it's good to see that greater community awareness and acceptance of the 'baby blues' is helping previously isolated women to seek and receive help.

Perhaps Fiona's greatest achievement is that she makes the reader feel normal, the goals attainable and the outcome positive. What better message to give a woman—you are good, you are healthy, you can be what you want to be.

This is a necessary book. It is warm, real and accessible. *Fit and Fabulous for life after babies* is an essential guide for all women before, during and after pregnancy.

VIJAY ROACH
Obstetrician and Chairman
The Gidget Foundation
www.gidgetfoundation.com.au

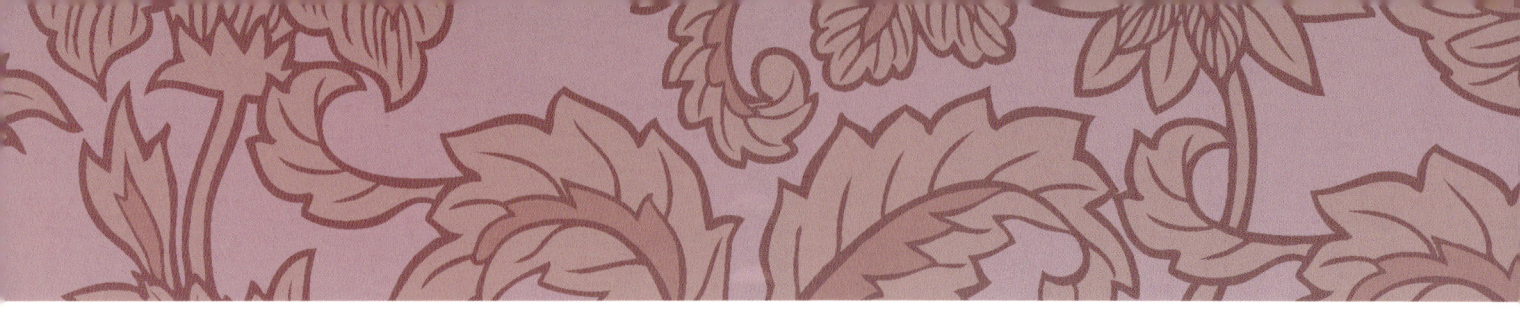

CONTENTS

Foreword	v
About the author	viii
Acknowledgements	ix

INTRODUCTION: SURVIVAL OF THE FITTEST

It's all about you!	3
If you fail to plan, you plan to fail	4
The program: keeping it real	6
How this book will work for you	9

PART I MIND POWER

1 Exercise your brain — 13

Kick bad habits	13
Clean up your environment	14
Strike a healthy balance	15
Don't rely on motivation	18

2 Stress less — 21

Put yourself on the payroll	22
The Supermum syndrome	22
Take a break . . . before you break	26
Stay positive	26
A healthy dose of reality	27
The K.I.S.S. philosophy	30
Go forth and conquer	31

3 Plan to succeed — 33

Step 1: Prioritise	34
Step 2: Time-saving strategies	35
Step 3: Schedule for success	39
Step 4: Start now	42

PART II ENERGY TO BURN

4 Energy balance and metabolism: Don't fight the system — 45

Diet is a four-letter word	45
What is metabolism?	46
Kilojoules and fuel	48
Body composition	49
The effect of body composition on metabolism	51
The energy equation	51
Fuel sources	55
Fuel preference and weight control	63

5 Food for body and soul — 65

Do not diet because . . .	66
Positive eating for good nutrition	67
Your body is a temple—treat it well	75
Check food labels	79
Portion control	80

6 Food for your lifestyle — 85

The food diary — 85
Purge the pantry — 88
Hitting the shops — 92
Meal inspiration — 93
Low-fat, 'light' and diet foods — 100
'My kids won't eat that!' — 102
Into the kitchen — 103
Pulling it all together — 104

PART III MOVE IT AND LOSE IT

7 Facts about fitness — 109

Why Exercise? — 109
What is fitness? — 109
The F.I.T.T. formula — 114
Don't forget to stretch! — 128
The pros and cons of joining a gym — 129
Home equipment to get you moving — 130
Setting fitness goals — 134

8 Exercising in pregnancy — 137

Stay hydrated during exercise — 140
Nourish yourself — 140
Your exercise plan — 143

9 The first trimester after birth — 153

Keeping it simple — 153
How to use the exercise tracker — 154
The first 24 hours: Your exercise plan — 155
The first six weeks: Your exercise plan — 159
Weeks six to 12: Your exercise plan — 164
Plan B — 171

10 The second trimester after birth — 173

Your exercise plan — 173
Plan B — 179

11 The third trimester after birth — 181

Your exercise plan — 183
Plan B — 187
When your nine months are up — 187

12 Beyond basics: Training with equipment — 189

A note on the exercises — 190
Your exercise plan — 190

Keep up the good work! — 197
Index — 198

About the author

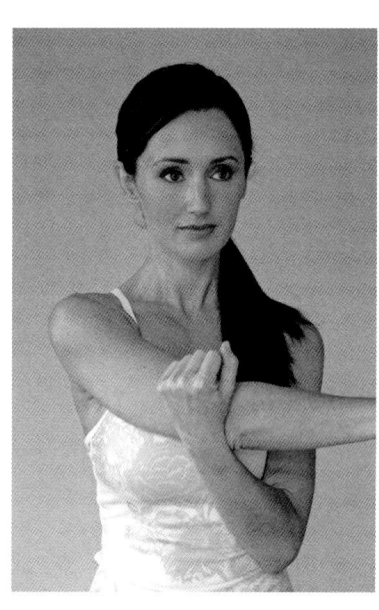

FIONA THOMAS HARGRAVES is an exercise scientist, nutritionist and mother of two. She studied her Bachelor of Science (Exercise Science) at the University of Southern California in Los Angeles and a minor in journalism at San Francisco State University, then interned as a clinical exercise physiologist at Scripps Memorial Hospital in San Diego. Fiona returned to Sydney for a post-graduate research fellowship at the Children's Hospital Institute of Sports Medicine at Westmead, where she co-authored *Pediatric Fitness*, and was a University lecturer in Human Movement before retiring to write and raise children.

A committed fitness professional since 1990, Fiona has considerable industry experience, including pediatrics, post-natal and corporate health; as a personal trainer 'to the stars' and an international presenter, and a group exercise instructor in Australia and the USA. Fiona writes for a London magazine and has appeared several times on Sunrise. She is completing a Master of Human Nutrition, speaks fluent French and studied landscape design for fun. Fiona lives with her husband and children in Sydney.

Fiona and her husband, Ben, support the following charities:

THE GIDGET FOUNDATION, which raises awareness of post-natal depression www.gidgetfoundation.com.au

THE HUMPTY DUMPTY FOUNDATION which supports children's hospitals www.humpty.com.au

Acknowledgements

Thank you to Publishers Annette Barlow and Catherine Milne who believed me when I said I could write this book and for pressing ahead with this project no matter what else they had going on behind the scenes . . . and to Matt Hoy who pointed me in the right direction.

Thank you to the Senior Editor Joanne Holliman who pulled it all together so efficiently, co-ordinated a superb creative team and was a delight to work with. I'm very grateful for Katri Hilden's skilful editing—she cut when I could cut no more—and for the proofreading done by Clara Finlay who caught everything I missed.

Thank you also to Liz Seymour whose brilliant design work made a stunning book out of a very plain manuscript. I am also very grateful to have had the opportunity to work with Katrina Crook whose beautiful photography brought the book to life and Lynn Wheeler whose make-up magic made me look like I actually had some sleep that week!

My gorgeous models Catherine Taylor and little Oliver; thank you for being wonderfully accommodating, for looking just amazing and adding so much to this book.

To Dr Vijay Roach, I greatly appreciate your kind foreword and support of this book but even more, your care and support while I had my babies.

Thanks to my lovely friends and sisters who are always a source of insight and often a supply of test subjects. And to my mother, Marlene Thomas, and my friend Sharon Fichardt for help with my children (and even the dog!) whenever I needed it; I couldn't have done this without your help.

Thank you to my parents Richard and Marlene Thomas for always encouraging me to do whatever I wanted and making sure I loved learning enough to never stop.

Thank you most of all to Ben, Caitlin and Lachlan for putting up with me being glued to my laptop and taking work on holidays . . . even when no-one else is allowed to. And thanks to Ben for his constant encouragement and support of every idea I want to explore, always believing in me and working harder than anyone I know.

FIONA THOMAS HARGRAVES

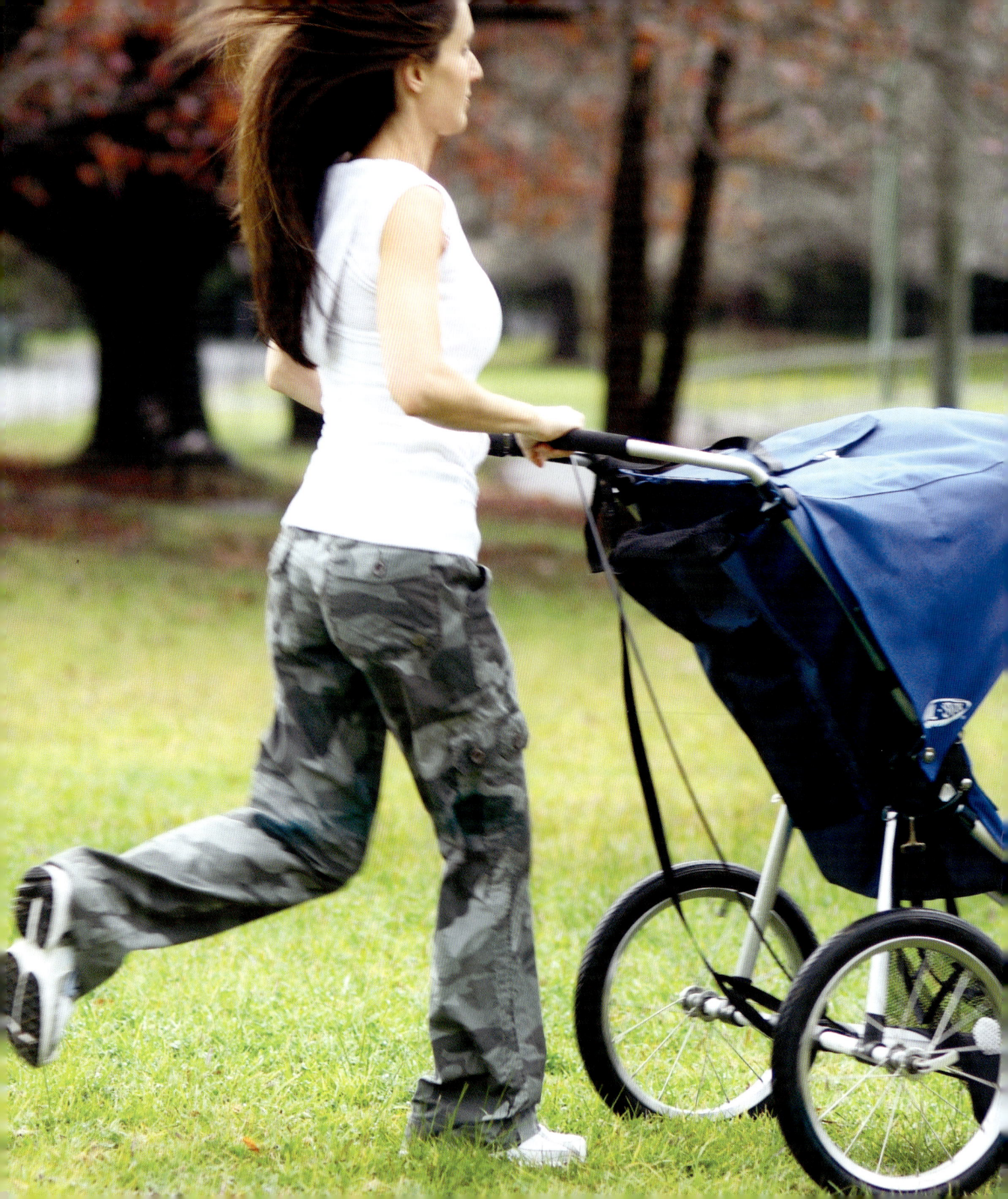

Introduction: Survival of the fittest

It's 2.16 a.m. The toddler had a bad dream and woke up the new baby who had just fallen asleep after 45 minutes of screaming. Now he's screaming again. If he's awake he thinks it's time to eat, but it's only one hour since his last feed and your badly cracked nipples are just not willing to negotiate a snack at this point. You've worn the same pyjamas for 36 hours straight. The last time you slept more than three hours was the night before the night before last, which explains your appearance and your mood. Your last three meals have been breakfast cereal straight from the box. You have stabbing pain in your back, your head is about to explode and you can't take anything strong enough to help because you're breastfeeding. Your partner is away for work for a week and everyone keeps saying, 'Oh, poor hubby, having to travel for work so much . . .'

If you haven't had the baby yet I don't want to ruin your romantic notions of motherhood. On the whole it will be fantastic, but directly after the event, most normal women probably feel more like a 'slummy mummy' than a 'yummy mummy' until they get it all together. What they don't tell you in the pregnancy books is that Hurricane Baby is about to hit you and the ensuing chaos can leave you in shock.

> 'A mother; 24–7 on the frontlines of humanity . . . are you man enough to handle it?'
>
> Maria Shriver

Don't worry, this is just the initial adjustment period and you will make sense of it. However, your life will never be the same again and this is an extraordinary and wonderful thing. If you're like every mother there ever was, there will be times when you think, 'What have I done?' But no matter how much you loved your former life and how crazy things become with your new life, you won't ever want to go back because of the amazing, tiny person who fills your days (and nights). You can become the eye of the storm: the chaos may still exist all around you but it will of course be organised chaos.

And you—well, you will be fabulous, fit and up for the job!

Job description of a new mother

WANTED: Kind lady to tend to every need of a very small person with inability to communicate effectively or do anything at all. This is a live-in position, 24 hours, 7 days. No holidays, sick leave or sitting down to rest.

EXPERIENCE: Not essential but would really, really help.

FORMAL QUALIFICATIONS: Not currently available in this field.

QUALITIES REQUIRED: Patience of a saint, psychic-quality intuition, patience, ability to perform under pressure with little sleep, patience, perseverance, willingness to deal with excrement and regurgitation on a regular basis, patience, ability to tolerate screaming for extended periods, ability to sacrifice own needs when necessary. Uniform of pyjamas, no make-up or glamorous hairstyles.

REMUNERATION: No monetary compensation, reward in kind only.

Nothing and no-one can *really* prepare you for this job. It is just one of those things that need to be experienced to be fully understood. Even those of us who attack the role head-on, armed with everything ever written or researched about babies, are still speechless the moment we meet our own baby and realise she is coming home with us for good.

Then you fall in love with this tiny person, and no matter what they do to you the love is eternal. And they will test you on this countless times a day at any age, yet still you realise that this is without doubt the most important job in the world. So, we know it's hard, and we know it's worth it. Now for you—what are you worth?

IT'S ALL ABOUT YOU!

There is nothing wrong with wanting to look good, or like you did before you had babies. It is not vain; on the contrary, it can be a fantastic boost at what is often a stressful and confusing time. This is the whole philosophy of the successful 'Look Good Feel Better' program for cancer patients, and it really does work. Think about it: how do you feel when you've got a great blow-dry, flawless make-up which makes you look fresh and natural, and you're wearing your favourite outfit, impeccably pressed, which enhances you in all the right places? You feel ready to conquer the world! Compare this to a day when you have barely had time to throw on trackie pants over your PJs, let alone think about a shower, your hair is tangled back in a nest-like bun and your skin is bare, dry and sprinkled with pigment and pimples from hormones . . .

We've all seen celebrity yummy mummies in glossy magazines, with infinite budgets to fund excessive pampering, but there is a *real-world* version of the yummy mummy. You'll see her at the park, the beach, the shops. She doesn't look like she's had a baby at all, let alone an armful of them in a few years! She is glowing and seems to have endless energy and enthusiasm for her role as a mother as well as for her other interests, friends and even jobs. You wonder how on earth she does it all with a newborn and a toddler or two running around . . . She is fabulous!

But it's not just about how she looks—she'd rather be a sane mum than a Supermum; she is not a martyr and asks for help or time out when she needs it. She is not a perfectionist and does not expect anyone else to be either. She does not feel that any aspect of motherhood is a competition, so she can relax and have good friendships. She has learned to compromise and prioritise and is prepared to let things slide if they don't really matter. She is optimistic about her abilities, has goals and is committed to doing the best job she can in her particular circumstances. She makes an effort to look after the minder of her children—herself!— as well, and as a result is healthy, fit to do the job and has an energy and confidence that others notice.

> 'An objective without a plan is a dream'
>
> Douglas McGregor

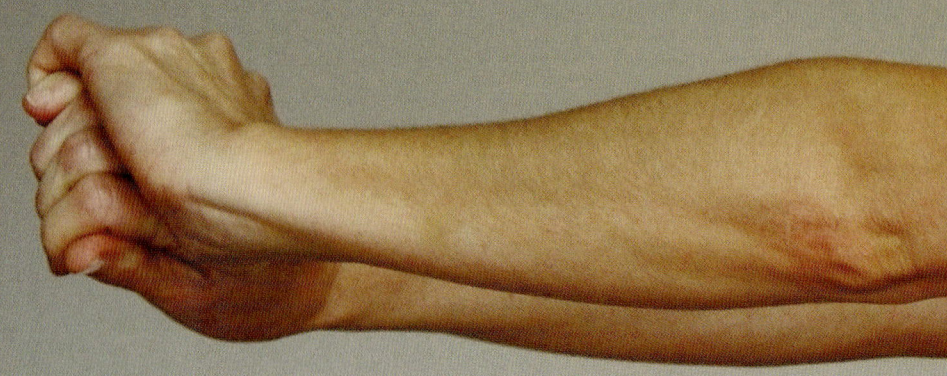

IF YOU FAIL TO PLAN, YOU PLAN TO FAIL

It's easy to tell a mother to make herself a priority, but anyone who has been a mother for more than a day knows this is extremely hard to do . . . unless you plan for it, prioritise it and make it happen.

Fit and fabulous mums aren't born with their babies and they're not made of wonder pills or meal-replacement shakes; they are built one plan at a time. If you ignore your health as the natural preoccupation with a new baby sets in, you'll wake up one day in a body you don't know and don't like, with a lifestyle to match. And it can then become difficult to turn the situation around as there seems so little time to achieve even the bare minimum every day. Another problem is that gaining 'baby weight' can become a vicious cycle, which compounds with subsequent pregnancies. Suddenly that extra five kilos from the first baby has turned into an extra 17 kilos, a bad back and shredded stomach muscles after the third baby, unless you do something about it.

You must make a plan or you will fall by the wayside!

I like to call it Plan B (for Baby). Plan A is how you would look after yourself if you had no-one else to care for. It is the optimal plan which would work perfectly if you had plenty of time and the inclination to do it. Plan B is what you will actually *be able to do* as a mother and stay sane. The objective is to plan ahead and then implement on autopilot so you don't have to think about it. It's scheduled in and when the time comes, you don't have to decide *what* to do or *whether* to do it—you can just do it. If you put 'must get fit' on your 'to do' list with no real plan, it won't happen because your focus will be

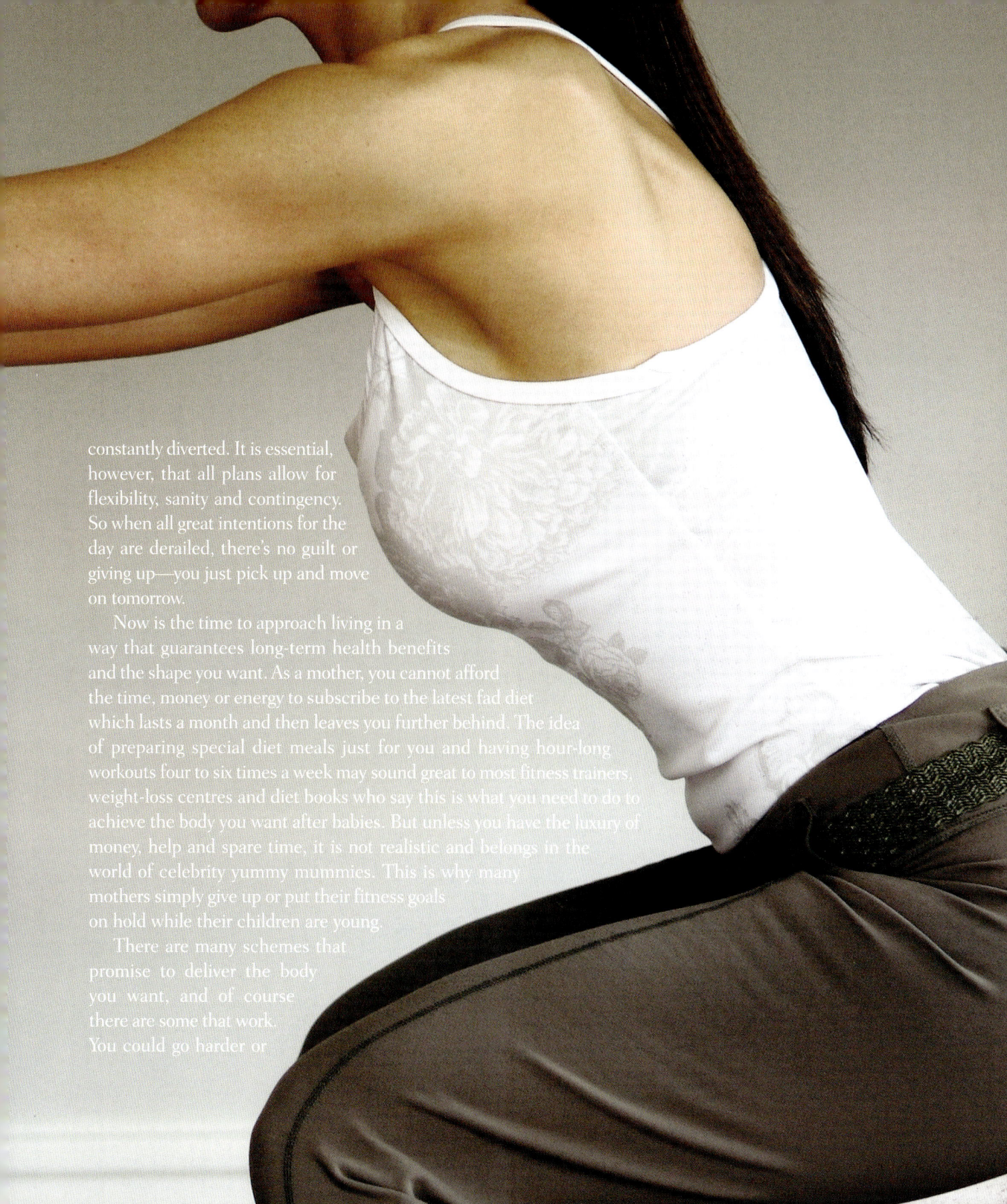

constantly diverted. It is essential, however, that all plans allow for flexibility, sanity and contingency. So when all great intentions for the day are derailed, there's no guilt or giving up—you just pick up and move on tomorrow.

Now is the time to approach living in a way that guarantees long-term health benefits and the shape you want. As a mother, you cannot afford the time, money or energy to subscribe to the latest fad diet which lasts a month and then leaves you further behind. The idea of preparing special diet meals just for you and having hour-long workouts four to six times a week may sound great to most fitness trainers, weight-loss centres and diet books who say this is what you need to do to achieve the body you want after babies. But unless you have the luxury of money, help and spare time, it is not realistic and belongs in the world of celebrity yummy mummies. This is why many mothers simply give up or put their fitness goals on hold while their children are young.

There are many schemes that promise to deliver the body you want, and of course there are some that work. You could go harder or faster if you're so inclined, but this book is for real mums who live in the real world, mums who will barely count crunches, let alone calories.

This book will help you achieve an optimal lifestyle *for you*. It will help you make the plans and then follow through to reach your goals.

THE PROGRAM: KEEPING IT REAL

Even though they may have personal trainers, chefs, nannies and housekeepers, I pity the celebrity mums who face media pressure to snap back into perfect form immediately after babies. The program in this book is not one which promotes getting back into shape in record time. New mothers already have enough stress, and intensive, quick-fix programs only set most women up for failure.

Regimes which are too intensive are unrealistic; they are not only unsustainable, but are often unhealthy and work against you in the long term. If you've ever been on a diet you may have experienced the mess dieting makes of your metabolism. During pregnancy, your metabolic rate is increased somewhat because your body is creating another person. The worst thing you can do after your baby is born is ruin your metabolism with a crash diet. There are many factors contributing to your metabolic rate, and severe energy restriction is the surest way to slow it down again and gain weight in the long term! And if you're breastfeeding, a severe diet and exercise program is difficult to sustain and can be unhealthy for you and baby.

Being overly concerned about pregnancy weight gain and obsessed with losing it afterwards is physically and emotionally detrimental. You may want everything back to normal as quickly as possible after the baby, but setting unrealistic schedules and goals will only lead to stress, disappointment and, most likely, ultimate failure. And you'll be miserable in the process!

If you've struggled with excess weight in the past, you may view pregnancy either as a serious weight risk or a free-for-all. I've seen both situations; the former leads to unhealthy energy restriction during pregnancy to control weight gain, and the latter results in excessive weight gain which is hard to budge after the birth. Both of these situations are problematic and it takes serious changes in attitudes and behaviours to adopt a healthier lifestyle for mother and baby.

This is a time to enjoy your new baby, and if you commit to looking after *yourself* as well, you can get back in great shape in a stress-free way.

Since it took nine months to get out of shape, it is reasonable to take nine months to get back into shape. I like to set this as a maximum time frame. It is kind and realistic and the biggest benefit is that it won't turn your life upside down (the baby already has that one covered!). If you have a caesarean, a complicated birth or a sick or particularly difficult baby, then allowing up to 12 months after the birth to get back into shape is reasonable. Your goals and results will also be influenced by the shape you were in before having the baby. I have trained women into better shape *after* babies than before, simply because they have committed to a healthier lifestyle than they'd ever had.

The nine-month time frame is not just about losing pregnancy weight. Your body also needs time to recover. Bones, ligaments, joints, skin and muscles all change during pregnancy, and many other physiological, biochemical and hormonal changes are still in effect months after giving birth, especially if you're breastfeeding. For example, some women will not menstruate again for six or even up to 12 months after the birth. You can return to your pre-pregnancy size and weight but remain a different shape for a year—or forever—after babies. A stylish friend who had a wardrobe full of beautifully tailored dresses and fitted suits could never wear them again after having her four babies, even though she returned to the same size, because her ribs, hips and breasts seemed to be in different places.

The World Health Organization recommends a minimum of 18 months (preferably 24) between a live birth and a new pregnancy to ensure optimal maternal and infant health. This may not be so much of a concern in a country with excellent health care, but their recommendation does acknowledge the physical strain and recovery required after pregnancy.

This plan works because it's sane

I was revoltingly sick with severe 24-hour morning sickness (hyperemesis gravidarum) and was hospitalised and on a drip for nearly a month with both my babies. I lost more than 10 per cent of my body weight in less than three weeks. I was put on steroids and a serotonin blocker as I'm inconveniently allergic to metoclopramide, a common anti-nausea medication.

I was fit before I had the babies, but my metabolism was totally ruined in the first trimester (with an involuntary crash diet) and I lost practically

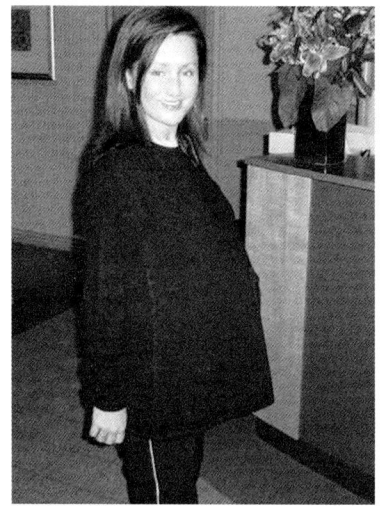

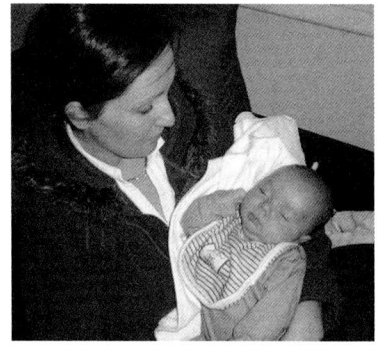

Yes this is me, the morning of delivery number two ... and then my beautiful son.

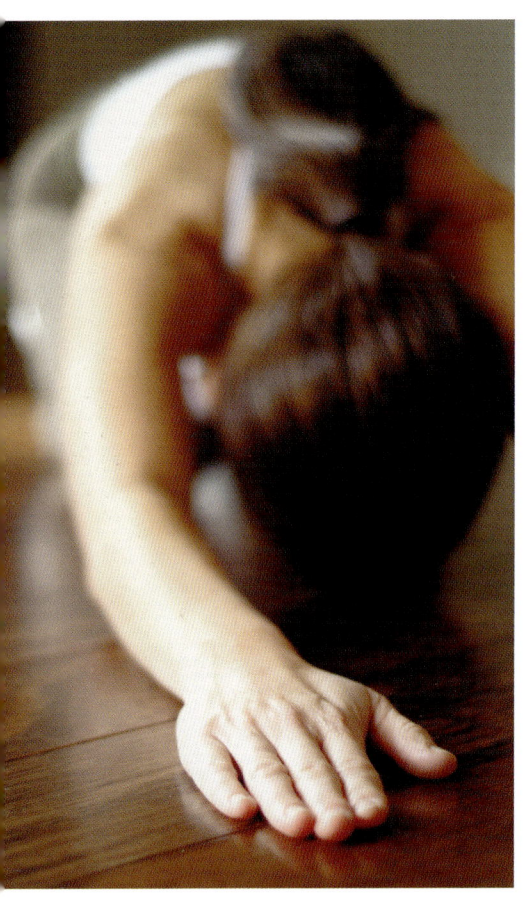

all muscle. When I could finally keep food down, I had to eat eight meals a day to get back to my starting weight and then make up for what I should have gained as well. But I was still too sick to exercise, so plenty of my weight gain was fat. Then, with the dreaded 'steroid bloat' and massive fluid retention, I put on about 17 kilos (net) each pregnancy. Being only 157 cm tall and having the skeletal frame of a pre-pubescent boy, that's a fair amount of weight, especially as my babies were both only around three kilos!

But all was not lost. I breastfed both my babies and I most certainly did *not* diet. However, I did eat positively, selecting foods that would provide adequate and long-lasting energy and nutrition for me and my milk supply without unnecessary empty calories. I focused on fresh, seasonal foods and I was not deprived—chocolate is always on my list, in moderation!

I concentrated on exercises to rehabilitate muscle groups such as the pelvic floor and torso for the first few weeks after the births. I soon started a little gentle walking and stepped up the exercise after my six-week check-up. Six months after the births I only had two to three kilos of extra pregnancy weight and I was still breastfeeding, so I had a few extra cup sizes in the bra to account for (I fed both babies for a year).

By nine months after the births I was back to my pre-pregnancy weight. A year afterwards I could tell I was still recovering in other areas. The skin on the stomach doesn't tighten up quite as readily—especially after more than one baby—and after breastfeeding, breasts can seem quite empty. But the body often finds a way to tighten a little more or lay some tissue back into the drained milk sacs after a year—give it time.

One step at a time

The last thing you need with a new baby is a complicated diet and exercise regime. The plan outlined in this book simply involves a series of smaller adjustments, which don't feel like 'going on' a special program and so are easily sustained. Basically all you need to do is replace less desirable habits with ones that are more conducive to your goals—but in a gradual way, so you're not obsessed with the exercise or what you must or must not eat. Before long you'll be eating in a positive way that energises and nourishes your body, and exercise will just become second nature. You will barely miss what you were doing before, but you will see the benefits, which will in turn motivate you to keep looking after yourself.

Your lifestyle is unique to you and will evolve as you direct it. No single nutrition and exercise prescription fits every woman's body and every baby's schedule. Beware of diets professing a 'sure fix for all': there are too many other variables such as physiology, genetics, hormones, schedules, commitments, abilities and challenges for any broadly prescribed regime to be universally successful or applicable long term.

I may not be presenting the quick fix many hope for, simply because it doesn't exist. But basically you should enjoy the approach outlined in this book, or at the very least not even really notice you're doing it, which is helpful in creating good long-term habits. But best of all, because you can sustain it, you cannot fail.

This is the *real* key to getting your body back into shape, and keeping it in shape.

HOW THIS BOOK WILL WORK FOR YOU

This book will help you create a lifestyle that will guarantee you stay fit and healthy while bearing and caring for children and beyond. The first part of the book helps spring clean your environment, behaviours and attitudes, which can too easily sabotage health and fitness goals, and also suggests strategies to help you manage your time and prioritise your health while juggling the demands of motherhood. Part II is packed with solid scientific information on why diets don't work, what to do instead to budge the baby bulge and how to get the best nutrition worked easily into each busy day. Then Part III gets you moving with the exercises every mother *needs* to do after pregnancy, those you'll *want* to do to get back into your pre-pregnancy jeans as well as a section to boost you beyond your former fitness levels when you're up for the challenge!

If you're not pregnant yet

Good for you, you're researching and planning ahead! The healthier you are now, the better you will cope with the physiological and emotional strain of 40 weeks of pregnancy, the delivery and recovery. You'll be well prepared for what's hopefully soon to come.

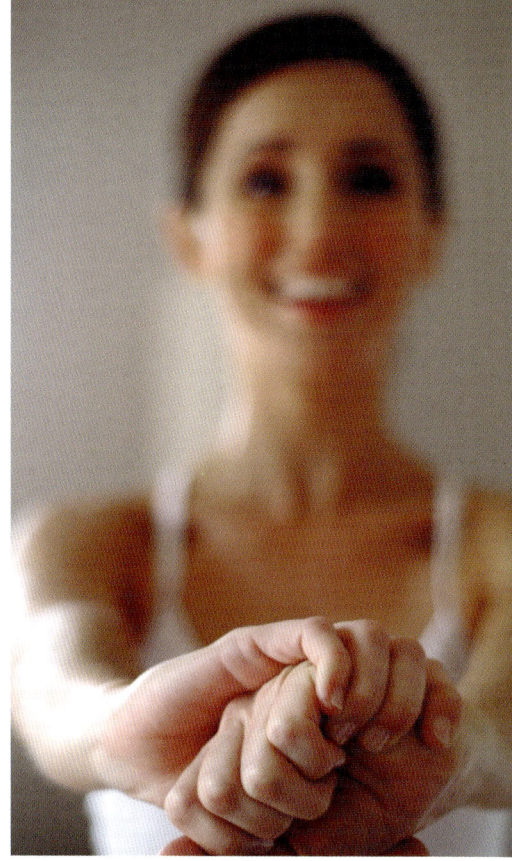

If you're pregnant

Well done! You've picked up this book at a great time, while you still have a chance to think about what comes next, make plans, set some goals, and keep yourself in good shape for the birth and beyond. After clearance from your doctor, start doing the exercises in chapter 8, then as soon as you deliver, get stuck into the other exercise chapters and work through each stage as appropriate, using the other chapters to consolidate your new lifestyle to come.

If you've recently had a baby

Congratulations! Even if you're a few months down the track, start the exercises at the beginning, but move through them a little faster to catch up to your current stage. Assess your lifestyle and look for areas in which you could improve your routines, nutrition and time management to promote optimal health.

If you've not so recently had babies

Good on you for realising that it's never too late to make changes and reach your goals, and for remaining open to new ideas and caring about your health. Depending on your current fitness level, you should be able to progress quite swiftly through the exercise trackers and make immediate modifications to your nutrition and lifestyle. All exercises are still relevant to any woman who has ever had a baby (as well as those who haven't!). Once you are competent with the basic exercises, focus on the recommendations for increasing the intensity of your workout so you will continue to improve.

At any stage before, during or after pregnancy, it is essential you have medical clearance before starting this program or any type of physical activity. Your doctor will be able to advise you of any precautions, considerations or modifications for your particular circumstances.

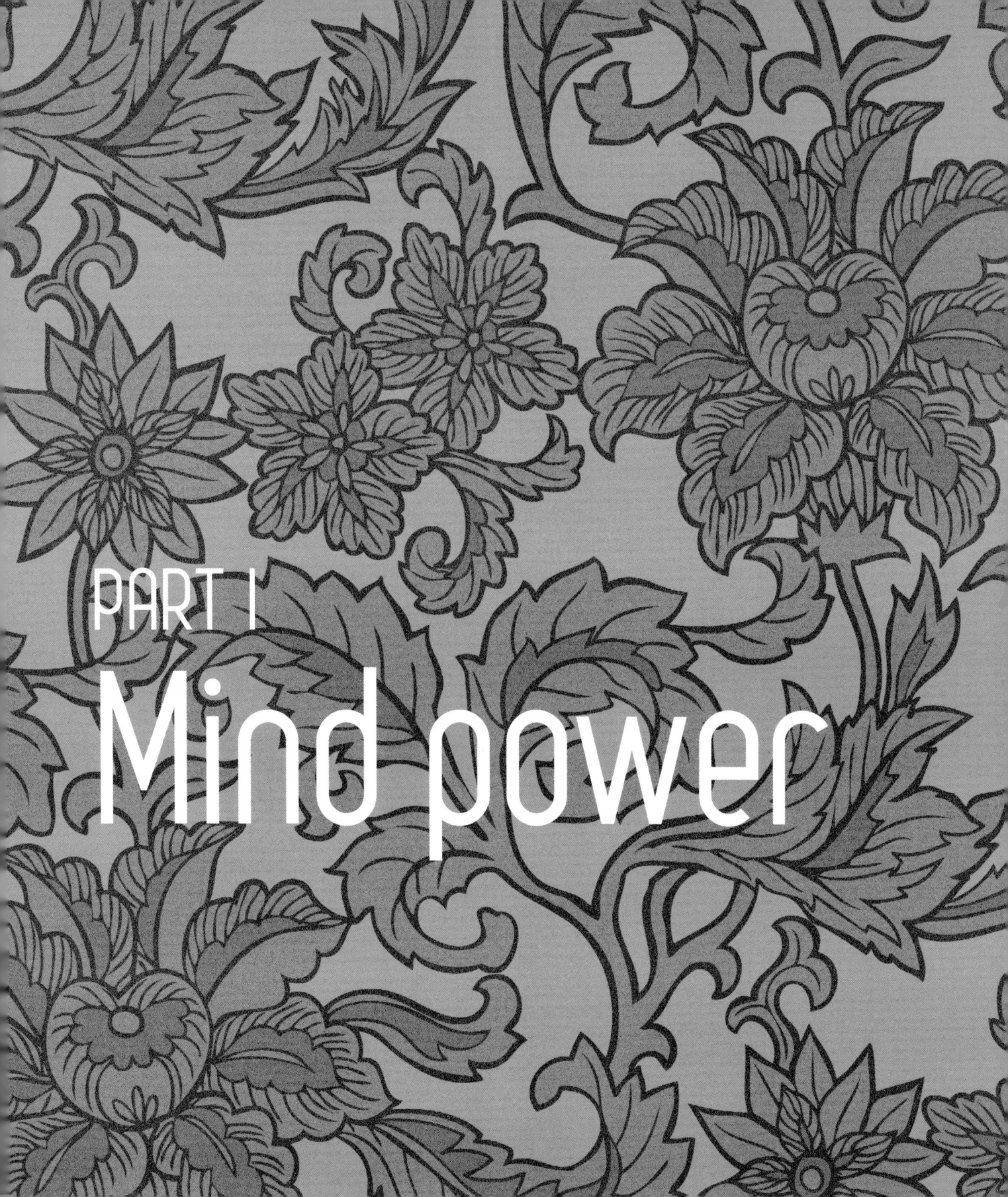

PART 1
Mind power

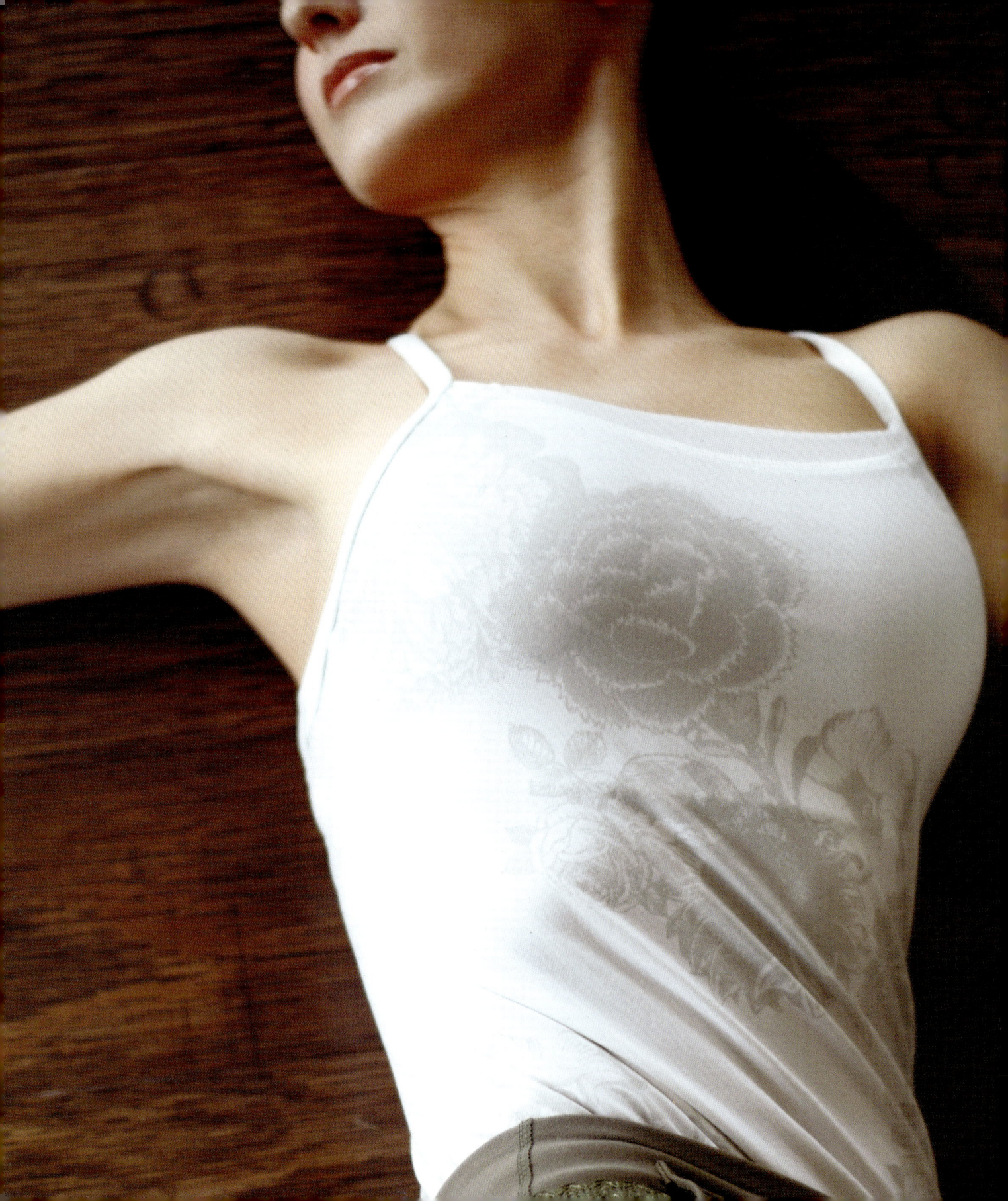

Exercise your brain

This is probably the most important section of this book. It is our behaviours, habits and attitudes that either stop us from or help us in succeeding at anything. Having the right information is important but doesn't guarantee we'll actually follow through. Most people know what to eat for optimal health and that they should exercise more, so why don't they just do it?

My friend Michelle sought the help of a nutritionist for guidance on how to clean up her diet to help her lose excess weight. When I asked about the session, she said, 'Well, I knew everything she told me. I know what I *should* be eating.' But the consultation made no difference as Michelle didn't commit to doing what it takes to achieve her goal.

The truth is that success ultimately lies with the individual. You can be given all the tools in the box, but it's up to you to use them.

Now just because you have to do this *for* yourself, it doesn't mean you have to do it *by* yourself. That's where this section comes in: your brain is the most important piece of fitness equipment you have.

KICK BAD HABITS

Our lifestyles are made up of what we do most of the time—in other words, a collection of habits. And our habits are formed by the behaviours we repeatedly choose to do and to which we become accustomed.

So, to change our lifestyle and habits, it's a matter of daily choices. We all have bad or less desirable habits. Some, like smoking, are blatantly obvious to all of us. Others we perform subconsciously in private, like standing at the fridge grazing before bed!

In identifying a path leading to better health or weight loss, it's important to be aware of the obstacles and to be conscious about your

Ready?

To get in shape, first shape up your head

Kick bad habits in favour of good ones: it's a choice

Create an environment that fosters success

The healthy mum's balancing act

Motivation is unreliable, so don't rely on it!

choices. A good place to start is the food diary in chapter 6. You may discover you are eating for reasons other than hunger (like boredom or depression) or that you have habits such as skipping meals and overeating later, or eating while watching TV or reading. Recognising habits that are working against you is the first step to changing them.

Many people claim not to have time to exercise, but seem to waste time elsewhere; it just comes down to priorities. We refer to time as though it were money. We talk of spending, saving, wasting, investing and buying time. If time were truly money, how would your investments pay off? Do you spend your waking hours mindfully, engaging in pursuits which matter to you and that improve your life and the lives of those around you? Or do you let time slip away, doing little that you want and always feeling you should be doing something? This is a habit.

By planning your days and knowing what you want to achieve, at least you'll have some direction. Regardless of whether it all goes to plan or not, step by step you'll start doing more of what you want and less of what you don't.

Once you've identified a habit you'd like to change, the best way to change it is to replace it with a more desirable one. The hardest way to get rid of an undesirable habit is to simply stop or go 'cold turkey'. Replacing a habit with a more desirable one is even more effective if you replace it with an *incompatible* one. For example, it may not seem significant that you finish baby's leftovers, but by the end of the week you may have racked up several unnecessary meals and kilojoules. One of many strategies for changing this habit is to simply put leftovers straight in the bin or the dog's dish—then it is highly unlikely you'll eat them! If you find yourself snacking at night after dinner or before bed, brush your teeth and rinse with mouthwash—most things taste pretty awful after that!

Find creative alternatives to replace, diminish, prevent, impede or end undesirable habits. Remember, habits are harder to break if you don't replace them with anything. You won't change overnight, but if you try a combination of tactics on a regular basis, it won't be long before you have a new, more desirable habit.

CLEAN UP YOUR ENVIRONMENT

Are you a product of your immediate environment, or is your environment a product of you? It's much easier to make better choices if the less desirable alternatives are not an option. If you are surrounded by junk food, there's no prize for guessing what you'll eat most of the time. If you spend a lot of time with people who make you feel bad about yourself, then your confidence will suffer. If you look for the easiest way to do everything—get food delivered, drive and park right at your destination, take the lift instead of the stairs—your everyday activity level could be practically non-existent.

To achieve the best lifestyle for you, plan for the best—for success. Keep healthy food readily available, put the walking pram and shopping bag next to the front door and put your car keys away. At mothers group, encourage the other mums to provide healthy snacks. When you eat out, choose restaurants which are generally healthier, so you won't have to 'use restraint'. Throughout parts II and III of this book I have provided tips on ways to make good nutrition and activity the easy choice. Remember, if you don't control your environment, it will control you.

There is much more to successfully achieving goals than just wanting. It is undeniably a journey; it's not a pill you take, or something you don't eat or don't do. Establishing a healthy habit takes repeated effort, fuelled by conviction and determination. Replace old habits one at a time with more positive actions and the old ways will decline and have less influence on your overall health. In other words, when the good outweighs the not so good, you're on the road to success.

STRIKE A HEALTHY BALANCE

Balance is essential to long-term, sustainable health, particularly when you have children. Don't think for a minute that if you can't manage the optimal 'Plan A' lifestyle you should give up altogether . . . doing something is *always* better than doing nothing.

Before having children, my gorgeous friend Sandra was a competitive cyclist. She was a serious athlete and prepared for races with determination and a strict diet and training regime, and was in fabulous shape of course. Sandra was one of the lucky ones when it came to pregnancy. She breezed through the 40 weeks, high on happy hormones, focused on healthy habits for herself and the baby. She recovered her pre-pregnancy shape quite quickly—but her challenges came in time.

Sandra has a classic 'all-or-nothing' personality. She has great focus and dedication to follow through and achieve, and won't commit to

> 'We first make our habits, and then our habits make us'
>
> John Dryden

something unless she is sure she will give it 100 per cent. The challenge, however, in being an 'all-or-nothing' type is that when babies come along, your focus is easily shifted to your new priority and you are left in the shadows. This is what happened to Sandra. After having two lovely baby girls 21 months apart, she became intensely focused on caring for them, which was natural and nurturing. But what about her? She ended up with poor eating and exercise habits and her body started to feel the strain of a new lifestyle of not-so-optimal habits. She didn't have serious weight problems, but she did ask me how to get back on track. She naturally wanted to address certain body parts, but I was more interested in her habits and what was going on in her head. We looked at ways of pulling focus back onto what she was doing for herself and scheduling in time to exercise and plan healthy meals.

Like a duck to water she was straight into it, and within a week showed me the most inspirational and flexible schedules and meal planners I've ever seen! It was almost like flipping a switch: Sandra was instantly back on track. Her children benefit from Sandra being organised and having lots of fresh food around, and they will learn from her example of being active and prioritising her health.

Sandra's story is not extraordinary; in fact it's quite ordinary. Most new mothers experience a period of intense focus on the baby. It's very natural, but the danger is that you can get totally caught up in only caring for the baby.

The key to doing it all is balance; realising you can do it all, but maybe not *all at once*. Knowing your priorities shows you how to direct your focus. When it comes to exercise, remember that Plan B is perfectly acceptable—and so much better than no plan at all.

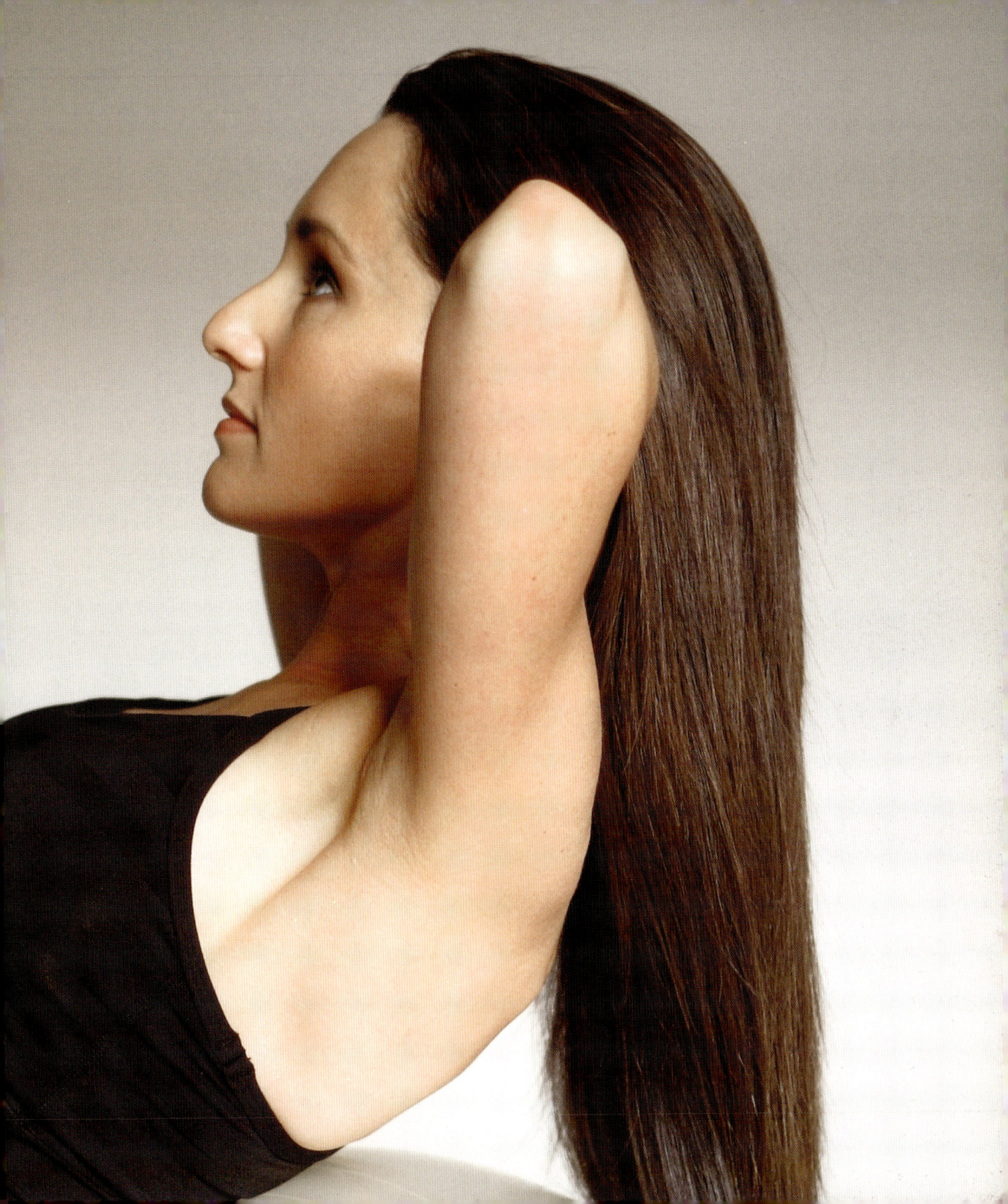

DON'T RELY ON MOTIVATION

A major problem with relying on motivation as an agent of change is that it flounders at the first slip-up or set-back. The problem is not that you skipped an exercise session or ate too many fries—a balanced life allows you that and more! It's what comes next: a downward spiral of self-defeating behaviour, characteristic to most rigid diets. If you perceive you have failed, your motivation will suffer, you will give in to thoughts such as 'Why bother, I've already ruined it!' and you're off the wagon again. If occasionally you accept two steps forward, one back, then as long as the net effect is moving towards your goal, you're winning.

In any endeavour, the first step is always the hardest. Minimise excuses for not getting out the door for a walk. The laundry is not as important as your health, and nor are emails. Put your walking shoes next to the door. When it's time to walk, put them on and go outside. Now that you're out the door, you might as well go around the block . . . or further.

Action is the true motivator—try it. And keep doing it until it becomes a habit.

If the general goal of losing weight doesn't inspire you enough to get out for a walk, focus on something specific about the immediate task—something positive about going for a walk right now, today. You may recall that you always really enjoy the walk once you're out—the fresh air, the chance to clear your head or think, or listen to your iPod uninterrupted, enjoying the scenery in your neighbourhood. Perhaps you don't feel particularly good during exercise, but focus on how good you feel *afterwards*, adding another few kilometres to your weekly tally, then relaxing in the shower, feeling proud and strong, knowing you're on your way to a healthier life.

A taste of achievement can be addictive—so become an addict!

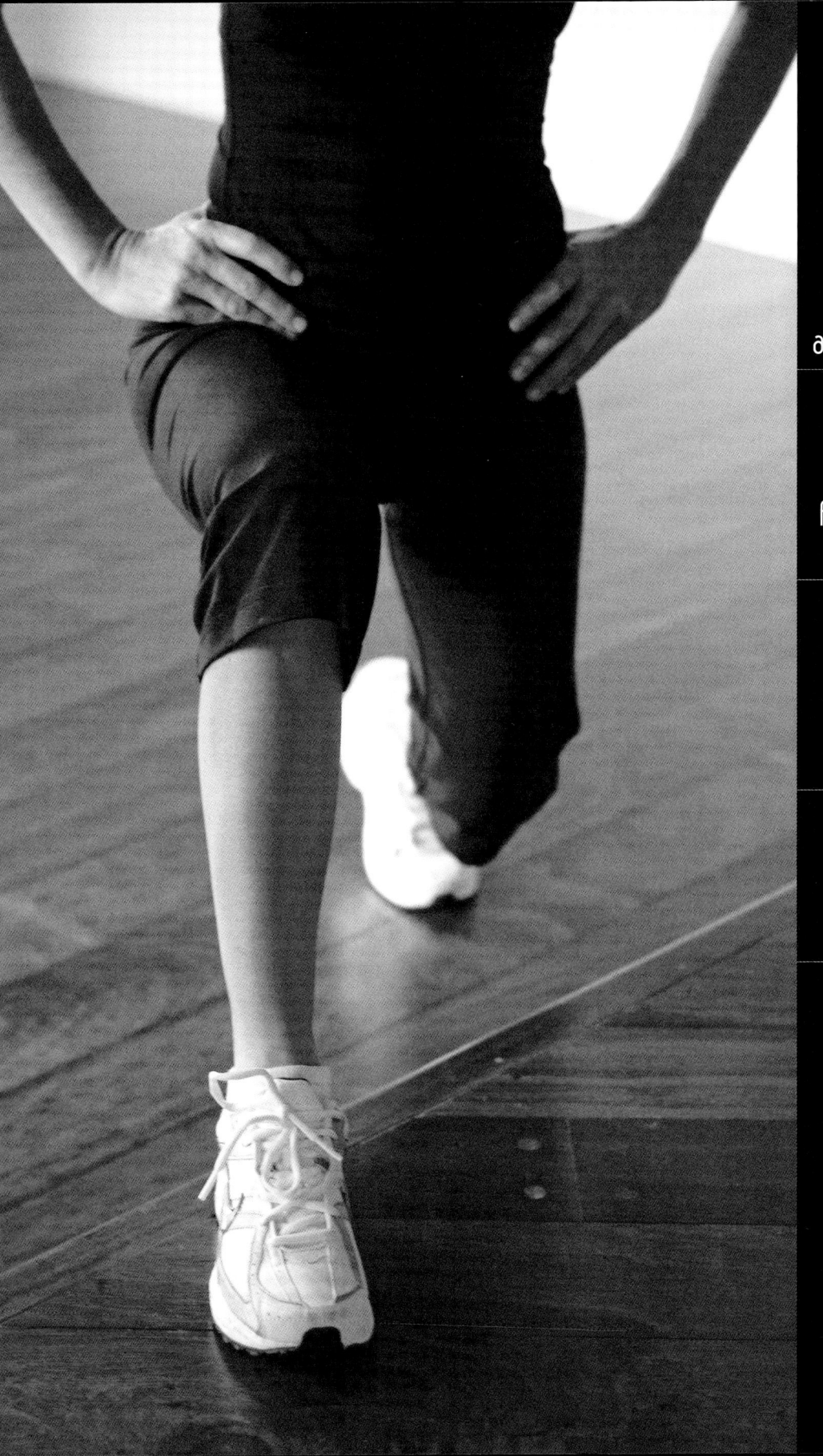

Action

Identify habits you'd like to change or that are working against you

Write a list of alternative actions, options or substitutes for these behaviours—then try them

Check your priorities: what do you ignore entirely and what do you obsess over? Balance it out

Don't wait for motivation to strike—decide to take action, every time!

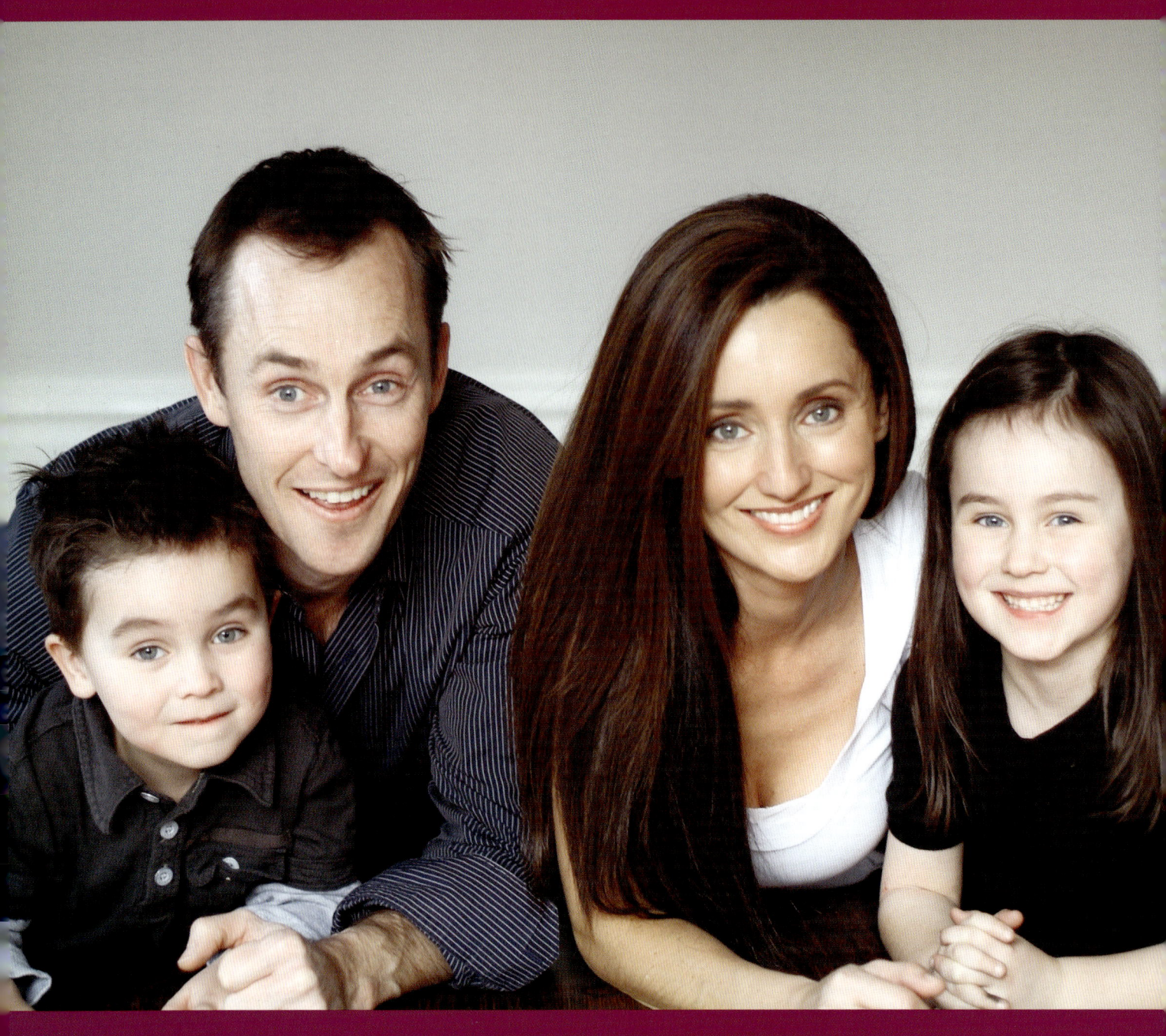

Stress less

Motherhood is wonderful but it can also be incredibly stressful, with its constant stream of new challenges. Physical stresses may include exhaustion, lack of exercise (and hence excess weight and poor fitness), poor nutrition, and muscle fatigue from the hard physical labour of holding and feeding babies or chasing and lifting toddlers. Emotional sources of stress are also common, such as feelings of inadequacy, low self-esteem, fear of failure in the role of mother, or difficulties adjusting from the 'adult world' to 'home-with-baby' world. I've been told that as a mother you never stop worrying—about everything. It's in the job description, so it's important to learn to deal with it and to keep things in perspective.

Feeling that you never have enough time and that everything is piling up is very stressful. Chapter 3 suggests practical ways to prioritise and manage your time so you can keep your health and fitness goals on track.

Having your head working against you can easily sabotage your best health efforts. As we saw in the previous chapter, your brain is the most important piece of fitness equipment you have. This chapter looks at some of the emotional stresses new mums face to help you get your head back on your side, as new mums already have enough obstacles to achieving their fitness goals. Just remember, a healthy mind and a healthy body go together.

Looking after yourself properly is the best gift you can give to your children. I don't mean obsessing about your appearance; I mean simply ensuring your body gets more of what it needs (such as good fresh food, exercise, relaxation) and less of what it doesn't (junk food, stress). It is not selfish; on the contrary, if you are dieting or obsessing about your weight or the chores you haven't done you'll be irritable, distracted and moody. If you can give your children a happy, healthy, energetic mother who feels

Ready?

Minimise unnecessary stress

Be kind to you

The truth about Supermum

Take time out

Keep it all in perspective

A quick reality check

great about herself, you will do the best job, naturally. And of course children learn more by example than any other way. When you value and look after *their mother*, your children learn self-respect and a sense of worth. Who wouldn't wish this for their children?

PUT YOURSELF ON THE PAYROLL

My philosophy in this book is more about nurturing than punishing regimes. My idea of nurturing doesn't equate to overindulgence, but simply means extending your nurturing attention beyond your offspring and giving yourself some too. It means cutting yourself some slack in the early days as a new mother and in periods of adjustment. It means being kind to you and being on your side rather than being your own worst critic. Be your own cheerleader instead—you have an enormous and significant job and you deserve congratulations every day! Remember, there is not only a new baby but also a new mother who has been reinvented, mind, body and soul—you! Get to know her, give her time to adjust and a chance to get in the groove.

How about putting yourself on the payroll and making sure you're taken care of too?

THE SUPERMUM SYNDROME

'You've got me, but who's got you?' Lois Lane asks Superman as he swoops through the air, rescuing her from a fall to certain death (*Superman: The Movie*, 1978).

Well, Superman can fly and has plenty of other superhuman tricks so he doesn't really need anyone to look out for him. But if you aim to be a Supermum, I hope you've got a back-up plan because there is no such thing. It's just an illusion the media uses to pump up their best-selling celebrities. And several years of being around mums with young children have taught me something about the competitive nature of the mother.

Through personal experiences and stories from my friends about their mothers groups, playgroups, friends and preschools it appears the Supermum Syndrome is rampant. Symptoms include ensuring everything *always* appears perfect, including children, house and the spread of freshly baked goods presented at a moment's notice. There are never stories to be told of a hard day or a trying night, of undesirable behaviour or of having had enough by the end of a long week. Everything is rosy, the kids are perfect, it's never a chore, there's never a fever or a fuss. And it's all done with a smile. Declarations abound such as 'No, mine don't have tantrums and the baby is already saying the alphabet as he learns to walk at six months!' Put-downs proliferate, masked as questions such as 'Oh, doesn't yours sleep through the night yet?' Of all fables mothers tell, this has to be one of the worst! In a certain group I attended for a while, every week the mothers were obsessed with comparing how the babies were sleeping. If yours hadn't done well that week you were made to feel like you didn't make the grade, as if your baby had a manufacturer's fault and you needed to trade her in for a new one!

Through my own informal polling, I have found that 'sleeping through' means anything from sleeping for a slightly longer stretch between feeds at night, sleeping from a 10 p.m. feed to a 3 a.m. feed or from 12 p.m. to 5 a.m. The only thing guaranteed with babies is that everything changes, good or bad, easy or hard, sleeping or not, it all changes—within the space of a day, a week or a month. Experienced mothers know to be thankful but not too hopeful when they get a good night's sleep, because it could all be over tomorrow night . . . and conversely, not to stress too much if they have the odd shocker.

Remembering that it is all ephemeral is a handy perspective when a windy baby cries for six hours straight, or you are going crazy trying to get the teething baby on a bottle (because your nipples are destroyed from biting) and toilet train the toddler at the same time. In a week, you will feel differently about it all, because the situation will have changed.

Perceived Supermums may turn out to be just that—a perception. Behind every seemingly 'perfect' exterior, there might just be a Desperate Housewife waiting to explode. I'm not saying that everyone is a raving lunatic, struggling to cope behind closed doors; it's just that everyone has hard days and more people will understand your experiences than you think. Women do not need to put more pressure on themselves and each other than they already bear!

> 'Often the worst enemy of mothers is other mothers and women must stop comparing themselves and their babies.'
>
> Vijay Roach

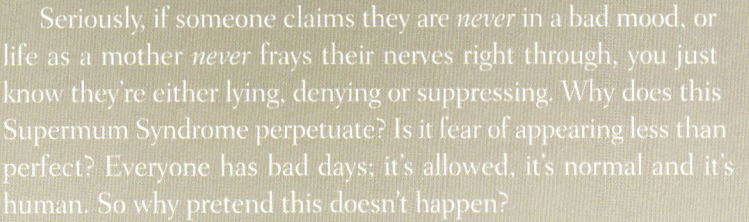

Seriously, if someone claims they are *never* in a bad mood, or life as a mother *never* frays their nerves right through, you just know they're either lying, denying or suppressing. Why does this Supermum Syndrome perpetuate? Is it fear of appearing less than perfect? Everyone has bad days; it's allowed, it's normal and it's human. So why pretend this doesn't happen?

My friend Kate seems the antithesis of a Supermum: she regularly calls me for what she labels her 'poor me' days. It's not that she's complaining, but she has a healthy appetite for the truth, 'telling it like it is'. She sugar-coats for no-one, and often just talking about the challenges of her days with four little ones helps her stresses evaporate and keeps her rational. The interesting thing is that she is actually a really great mum to happy, healthy children and is also fabulous. Her venting is an effective stress-management technique.

This is my idea of a super mum.

Every new mother needs a real support group as a trusted 'board of advisors'. They may be relatives, friends, neighbours, early-childhood nurses, your partner of course—anyone who has your best interests at heart, does not see you as 'competition', who listens and offers honest advice when solicited. Sometimes all that is needed to dissipate a stressful situation is a sympathetic ear, especially from someone who has probably had a similar day. Remember you're not alone and that although no-one's experience is exactly like your own, there are many who will understand.

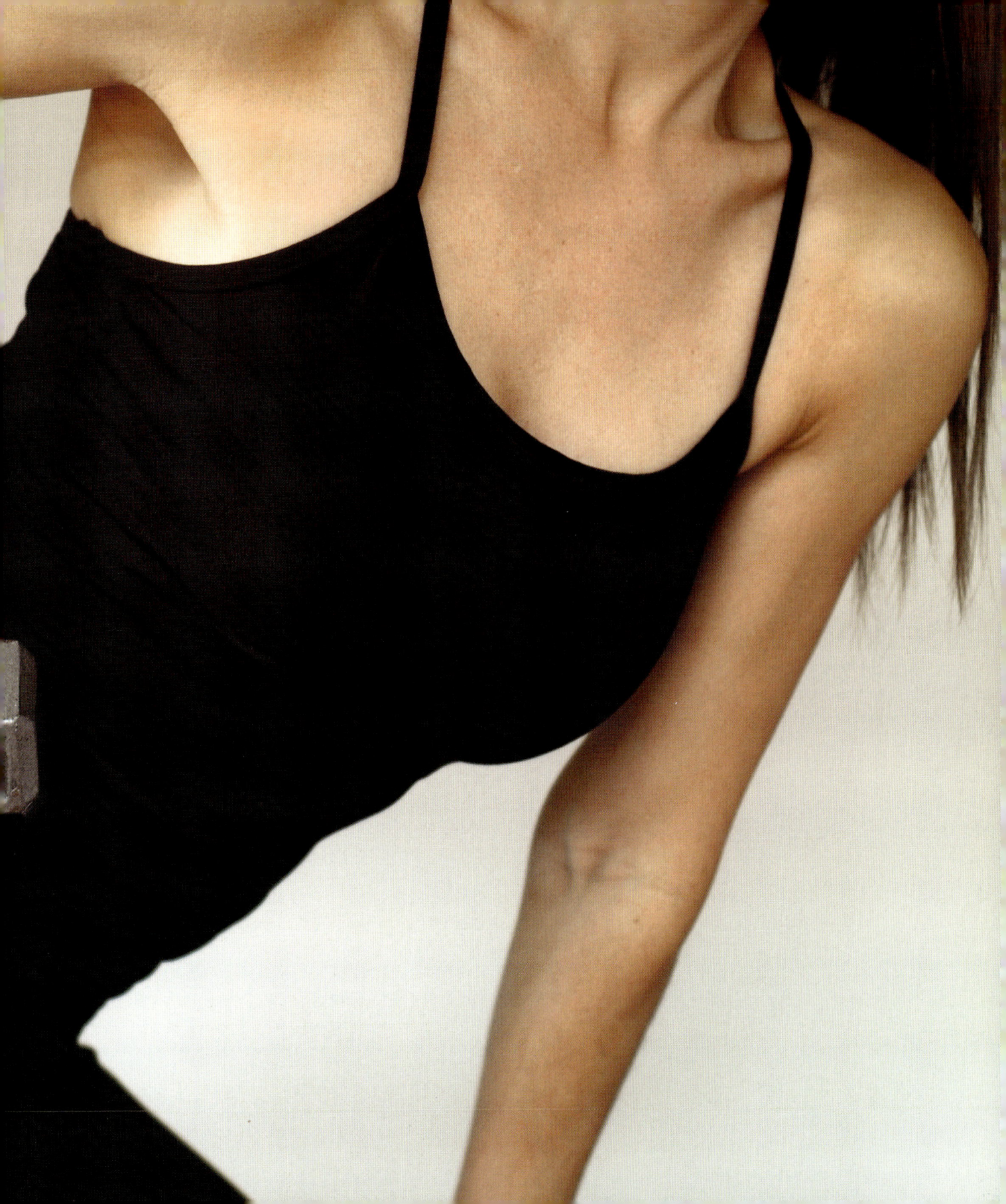

TAKE A BREAK . . . BEFORE YOU BREAK

It is a new mother's disease to think she cannot do anything for herself or ask for help—there is no other employ where one would indulge in such self-sacrifice. Recognise your limits, we all have them. Sometimes you have to say 'enough' and look after yourself as well . . . and take pleasure in life before your life gets the better of you. Your life doesn't stop when your child's starts. Include children in your plans: they *are* portable and will become enriched by you living a full life.

Taking a short mental break defuses the cumulative effects of stress. Do something you enjoy—or nothing at all!—for a little while each day. Make it a priority to relax and recharge by doing something you want to do, not because it's 'on the list'—watch a favourite movie, have coffee in good company or in peace, email faraway friends, read a light-hearted book or magazine just for fun, have a nap, take a bath, lie on the grass.

Exercise is one of *the best* ways to relieve all types of stress. It is a form of physical stress—but a good one! And the 'down time' or rest between training sessions is equally important as the exercise itself. It is during *rest* that the body recuperates and responds to the physical stress it has undergone by becoming fitter, stronger, better. Without rest, the body does not get a chance to repair the physical stress and immunity is compromised. The same is true of emotional stress.

STAY POSITIVE

Optimism is simply adopting an open mind and a positive, 'can-do' attitude. Being an optimist is a choice. It starts as a way of thinking or an approach, and leads to a behaviour—how you act or react. It doesn't mean *always* being happy no matter what's going on. Feigning optimism or blind optimism isn't real, doesn't help anyone and annoys many.

A healthy balance between realism and optimism will let you accept with peace that things will not always go your way, but allow you to keep trying, move forward and focus on your goals, because if you stop trying for what you want you'll definitely never get it.

If your new baby had a terrible day, week or month and you've totally ignored your exercise regime and survived on takeaway, chips and chocolate, don't dwell on it—all is not lost. Tomorrow is a different day—another chance to try, if you want it to be, or it can be the same again. But don't feel guilty—there will be plenty of opportunities for guilt as a mother. Let it go! Until a reliable method of time travel is available, you can't change what happened yesterday, but you can decide what happens tomorrow.

Negative thoughts inevitably enter your head some days. Suppressing or ignoring them won't make them go away, but addressing and rationalising them and putting them in perspective can help. For example, is it *really* likely that everyone thinks you look fat? No . . . they're either more worried about themselves or too distracted by your new accessory (your baby) to even notice your body. Chances are, your partner loves your curves and it probably drives him crazy that baby gets the good bits all the time. Just relax, stay positive and enjoy the amazing gift you've been given.

According to studies by Tresillian Family Care Centres, up to 70 per cent of women experience 'baby blues' lasting from days to a few weeks. Rely on your support group and surround yourself with positive people at this time. Optimism is as contagious as pessimism and I know which I'd rather catch. If the 'baby blues' persist longer than a few weeks and you can't get positive, see your doctor. Postnatal depression is a serious condition that affects about one in five Australian women. There are several treatments to explore and the sooner women seek help the better.

A HEALTHY DOSE OF REALITY

Setting goals is an important part of any fitness program. Daily, weekly and longer-term goals keep you focussed on what you've decided is important to you. Keep in mind that very specific plans are not generally easy for a new mum to follow. Your body may not respond to pregnancy in exactly the same way the second or third time around, especially considering you have other children to care for. Your post-pregnancy schedule will be much busier with subsequent children and your body may bounce back more easily the first time than the fourth.

No-one has your exact experience, your precise physiology, your mind or your life situation. You will frequently suffer disillusionment if you compare yourself to celebrities, models, friends or family, as you only ever know half their story—if that! Just compare yourself to your best version of you. Let go of 'perfect' and go for great, yummy, fabulous! Perfect does not exist. The pressure from the pursuit of perfection will make you quit when the outcome of your efforts cannot ever match your expectations. All you can do is your best; play the hand you're dealt, work with what you've got and be realistic.

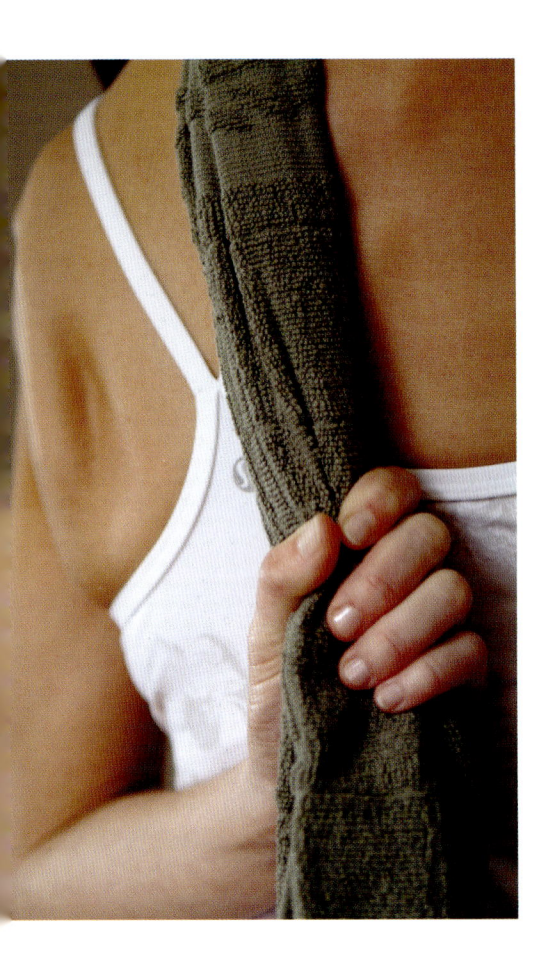

Being realistic is not a euphemism for accepting second best, it just means knowing your body, how it used to be, what it's been through and recognising that some changes are more permanent than others. There are inevitable changes during pregnancy and as a mother, so just concentrate on what you can control—your lifestyle. Undesirable habits take a long time to establish, and cannot be replaced with good ones overnight, so be patient.

Remember also that for a plan to work, it must suit your lifestyle, tastes and abilities. You need to evaluate changes and determine if they will work for you. It's worth giving anything a try, but if you won't enjoy something enough to sustain it, then consider an alternative to which you could better commit. There is always another way—it may not be the first choice, but it will do the job.

My friend Alana wanted to get back to her pre-pregnancy weight after baby number one before getting pregnant again; her deadline for 'going again' was approaching quickly and her weight loss hit a plateau with eight more kilos to lose. She knew what she had to do in terms of healthier eating, and was happy to walk regularly. However, no matter how much I insisted she try resistance training to really get her body going, she would not even entertain the idea. Alana tells me she's lazy. She hates exercise, especially if it's planned, structured or hard. But she is good at commitment, she is realistic and she's a smart girl who knows herself really well.

Alana knew, better than I, that a resistance-training program for her was about as useful as a pencil to a fish. She simply couldn't use it because the most important part of her wasn't able to: her head. So Alana just focussed on the modifications she could happily do: she ate well and walked most days. She didn't squander her efforts on other changes which, although more optimal, would have failed her. Sure, if she added resistance training her plan would be more efficient and produce better results more quickly. But she knew her limit and as a result was immediately well on her way to reaching her goals—and had lost a few kilos when she got pregnant again after less than a month. When you're a mum, the best-laid plans are always interrupted by baby!

I consider Alana's a great success story. Even though she wouldn't do everything I wanted, she was committed and did everything she promised herself. The lesson here is to balance idealism with realism. You may not enjoy or be able to do everything I suggest in this book, but give it a go and if something really isn't working for you, change it. The plans, schedules and new habits you'll form will keep you on track when your willpower wanes and motivation fades.

The key to lasting success is to avoid the all-or-nothing mentality. Avoid the pressure of thinking it's not worth the effort unless you can do it perfectly, dramatically, urgently.

Start right now, with what you can do, and just move forward. Your continued motivation comes from the rewards you feel and see as a result of pursuing an optimal lifestyle and of really living healthfully.

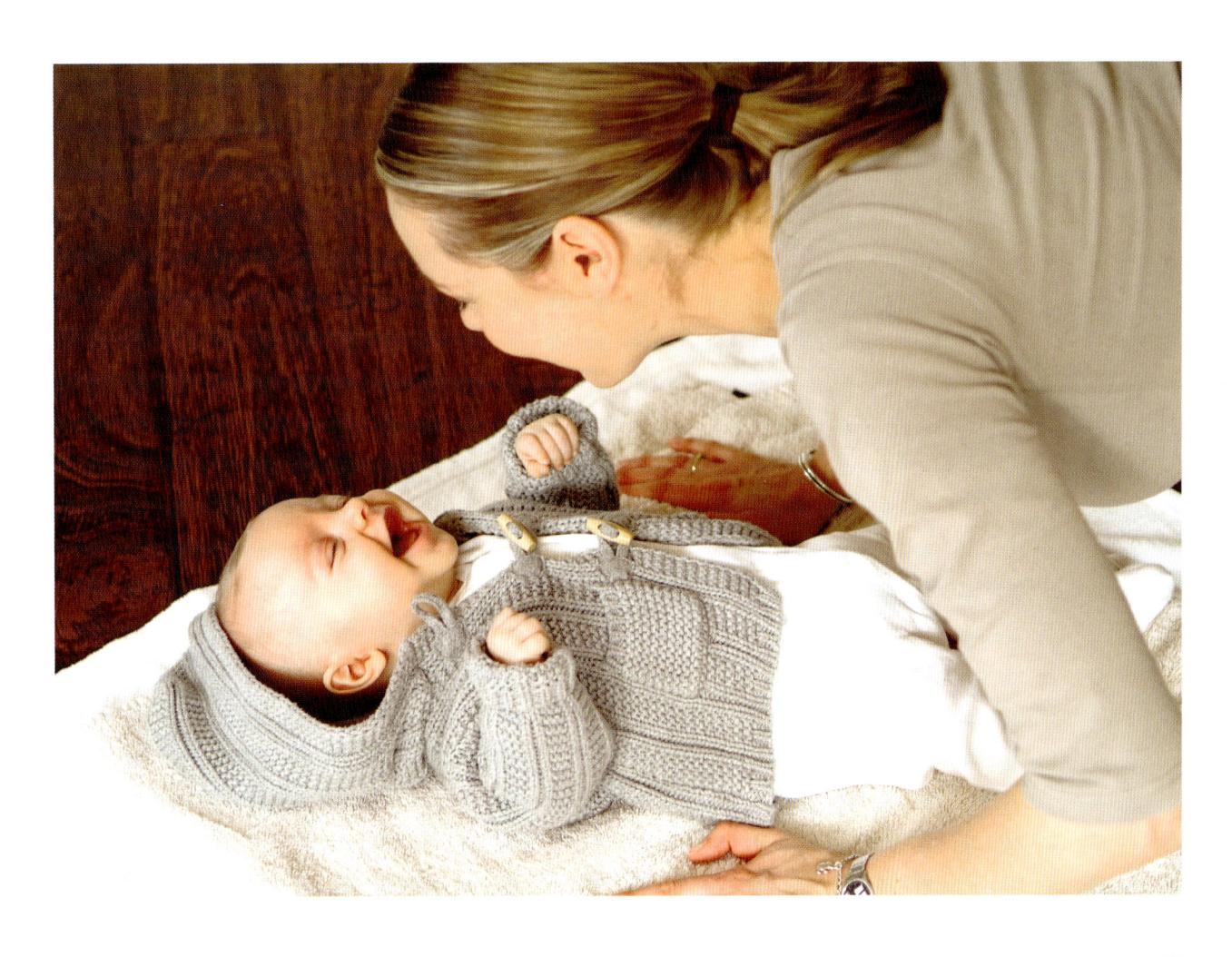

THE K.I.S.S. PHILOSOPHY

I am a firm believer in keeping things simple. Sometimes more is just more, and this is true when it comes to diet and fitness. I find that fitness regimes and their longevity are inversely correlated: the greater and more involved the regime, the more fleeting its existence. The best plan is always the most straightforward, realistic, convenient and therefore sustainable, which means results. The K.I.S.S. philosophy is the perfect mantra for busy mums: Keep It Short and Simple!

Let things slide a little. Prioritise what's important—people. Obsessive behaviour is destructive and draining for busy mums. Obsession over food, exercise, chores—it's all unnecessary stress. If you make a plan, decide it's worth it and commit to it. Agree to moderation and balance so you can enjoy your babies while they're young. You'll never look back and wish you had obsessed more about ironing or the kitchen sink. But you may wish you'd enjoyed your little ones more while they were tiny.

In planning your health goals, you are setting yourself up for success, but remember that you cannot change just by *wanting* to. You have to decide you *will do* what it takes, consciously determine how to do it and then commit to doing the work. Quite simply, have a plan and follow through with it.

Once you have the framework for your program and the tools to adapt it yourself, there is no need for expensive gym memberships or personal training sessions which you probably wouldn't have time for anyway. Determine what's right for you, and take charge of your own life and health. Once you know how to plan and manage your health, you can permanently avoid fitness fads and diet traps and successfully navigate the various stages of being pregnant, recovering, having subsequent children and beyond.

Although it may sound like a great challenge to really overhaul your lifestyle for good, consider how hard it is to live without optimal health. How hard is it to be overweight, tired, unfit or unhealthy? As Australian celebrity TV expert Dr John Tickell once said, 'If you can't put a little time aside now for recreational exercise, make sure you put away a lot of time later for illness.'

Bad habits are as cumulative as good ones. Doing nothing is as much a choice as doing something. You will reap what you sow, more or less.

GO FORTH AND CONQUER

There is always something out of the ordinary happening. Life is a journey which encompasses a huge range of experiences, from births and deaths to marriages and divorces, travel and moving, special occasions, starting a new job or studying, illness and stress. You cannot wait until there's nothing left to do to focus on your health, as that time may never come.

As outside factors change, adapt to them and do what you can, when you can. Listen to your body, be kind to yourself, know what is good for you and do it. It's never too late to live a healthy lifestyle and it will only ever help. Your body is a precious vehicle to get you through life. If you look after it appropriately, with balance, then you can enjoy all the richness life has to offer.

Action

Nip stress in the bud with exercise, regular time out and a positive attitude

Don't worry so much—worry feeds stress

Check your glass: is it half-empty or half-full?

Believe in yourself and what you want

Check your life for toxic influences and clear them all away

Mix exercise with good food, a little chocolate, a healthy dose of positive attitude and lashings of self-respect . . . shake and take daily!

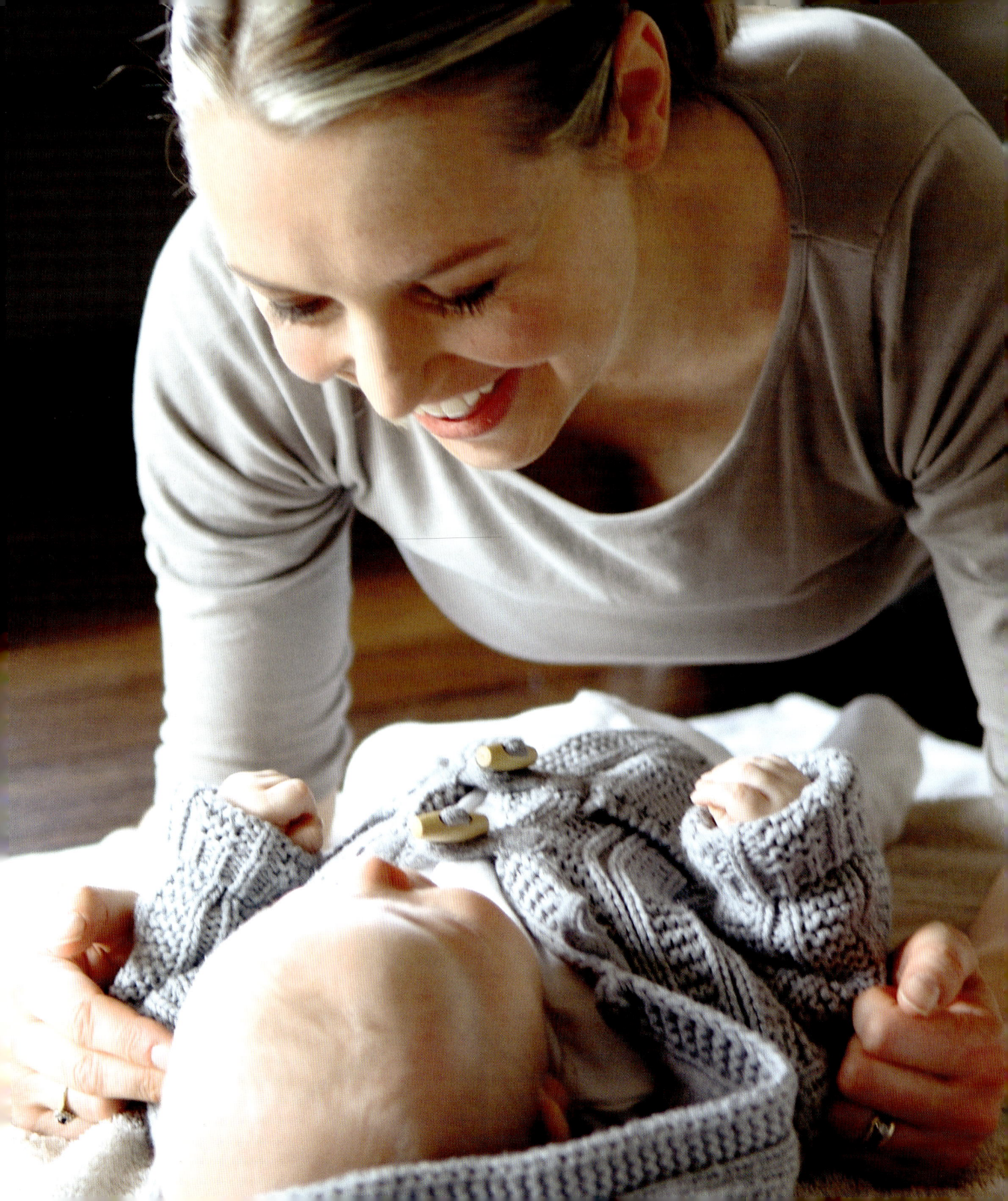

Plan to succeed

You're probably thinking the last thing you need right now is another project, but this one is not hard. In fact it's quite simple, and getting organised will actually give you *more* time.

You may have heard the saying, 'If you want something done, give it to a busy person'. Busy people are efficient because they become good at time management, planning and prioritising.

At the end of a busy day many mums look around and think, 'What did I really get done?' In the early days with a newborn, the endless feed–change–settle–feed cycle leaves you able to do little else, especially if you have other young children to care for. But as the weeks roll on you get into a groove and you can find some time for you, if you plan it. You will be amazed at how efficient you can become with a little scheduling. This does entail running a fairly tight ship, but with flexibility.

Mothers never stop. This job will consume all your waking and many of your supposed sleeping hours if you let it. But you do not have to sacrifice yourself to do a good job. Constantly being the martyr will not do your family any favours if you develop exhaustion, resentment and poor health. Of course your children are your priority, but your children also need and deserve a healthy, happy mother.

I've heard many mothers talk about what they'd love to do *one day* when they have time. Well the reality is, now that you're a mother, things only get busier! And if you don't make time for your health and fitness now, then you make time for sickness later.

Planning everything is the only way to ensure you manage time efficiently. Meals, shopping, work, cleaning, activities and exercise all need to be scheduled into your life. The only way to exercise regularly and make it a habit is to set aside a prioritised time. If you have a partner or friend who wants to walk or exercise with you, great! Making an appointment with someone else locks in a time and helps you commit.

Ready?

Think you can't fit it all in? Think again

Top time-management tips for busy mums

Organisation makes life run smoothly

Practical ways to prioritise and plan—step by step

Your time starts now . . .

STEP 1: PRIORITISE

Your life is yours to do with as you will. Don't lose sight of your passions or of what you always wanted to try. Keep these on the list. Be realistic about the different stages of life with babies—although some plans are temporarily on hold, never forget who *you* are. When the time feels right, take that tap-dancing class, renew your studies or pick up a brush and paint. You will be energised by the novelty, refreshed by the distraction and fulfilled by the varied experiences of life. But for now, look at what you really have to do and what you really *want* to fit into your week.

Write a list of all the things you have to get done and things you want to do, then rank them according to how important they are to you. Your list may include the following:

- caring for children, playing with children
- recreational outings with children—swimming, park, kindy-gym, dance/music class
- school or preschool drop-offs and pick-ups
- daily meals, cooking and eating
- grocery shopping
- sleeping
- social outings—mothers group, playgroup, coffee with friends, play-dates
- walking or other aerobic exercise
- strength and flexibility exercises
- work (from home or out of home)
- daily chores—cleaning the kitchen, general tidying, beds, laundry etc.
- freezer cooking
- weekly chores—bathrooms, floors etc.
- a recreational activity for you—a class, book club, coffee with friends, a date with your partner (remember those?)
- other 'you time'—go to the hair salon, take a nap, do nothing.

In compiling your list of priorities, never overlook the importance of sleep. Everything seems insurmountable when you're a walking zombie; every little request from baby crushes you like a whining 10-tonne weight. But a decent sleep makes you feel you can tackle the world and stay on top of things and this attitude is *the* best tool in the kit for a mother. According to the Black Dog Institute, lack of sleep and increased levels of fatigue lower emotional resilience for parents and can be a risk factor for postnatal depression.

We all need different amounts of sleep to function optimally, but in general eight hours is recommended. Okay, I know it's a rare luxury for new mums and you may function fine on five or six hours with a rest in the afternoon while baby naps. But do whatever you can to make up for sleep lost during night feeds. Recruit your partner for a night feed if baby will take a bottle. Get a friend or relative to take a fussy baby for a walk. A good nap just one afternoon a week can recharge you enough to go on for another week. Take advantage of the times when your partner is around (like on the weekend) to catch up on rest. Insist on one sleep-in a week if you can arrange it—one of life's most delicious luxuries! Prioritise sleep over things like laundry and even exercise if you're really tired in the early days.

Just sleep and eat well to keep your immunity strong, otherwise you risk getting run down and sick, which compounds fatigue. Your body recharges and repairs during sleep, and if you're not getting enough, you'll end up flat on your back—one way or another.

STEP 2: TIME-SAVING STRATEGIES

As you consider your priorities, determine where you could save time and what you could let slide. No-one can do 100 per cent of everything 100 per cent of the time and still be sane! The following section offers ideas on how to focus your efforts and use time more efficiently . . .

Meal planning

The most dreaded time of the day: late afternoon rolls into early evening, children are fractious, mum is no better, and the always-looming question arises, 'What are we going to have for dinner?'

A good friend sometimes phones about 5 p.m. to ask what I'm making, in search of inspiration. This is because I have the weekly dinner menu on a cafe-style chalkboard in my kitchen. I write it up after the weekly shop, and it's one of the highlights of my husband's week—he loves his food and likes to know what's in store—and the children also enjoy the 'specials' at the 'restaurant'! It's a bit of fun, but also really helpful for staying organised. And the most important part of the menu board is my disclaimer at the bottom, which reads: 'Chef reserves the right to change without notice . . . or to not cook.' It's a clause I exercise on a regular basis!

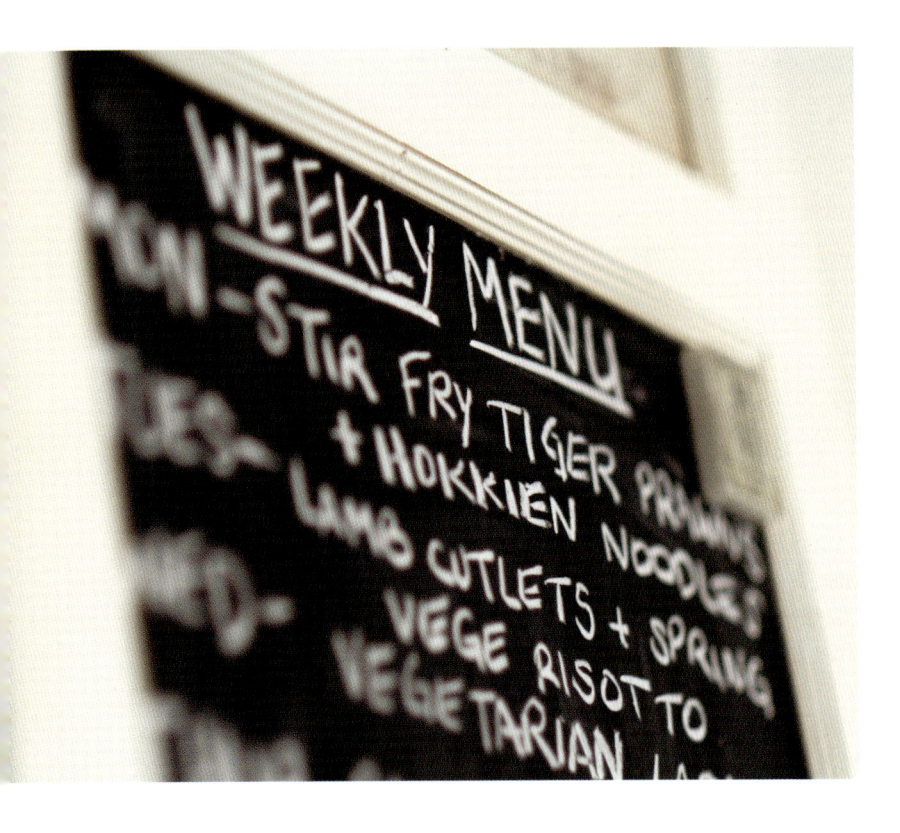

Dinner may be the only time when the family comes together during the day, so there's pressure to produce a substantial spread. But the last thing you want at the end of a busy day is more decisions about more food. Time, nutrition and budget can all be compromised by lack of planning. Chapter 6 addresses meal planning in more detail, including creating weekly menus, cooking in bulk to freeze or in advance, shopping lists, essential pantry, fridge and freezer items, and coming up with creative, simple and speedy meal solutions when there is 'nothing in the cupboard'.

Organisation

There is nothing like the feeling of a fully ordered environment. Things may look clean and neat, but if 'stuff' has been pushed under the couch, crammed in drawers and the cupboards are bursting at the hinges, full of clothes the children grew out of two seasons ago and toys they never look at, the house will be a total mess again in half a day. Then you spend the rest of the day stuffing it all away, just to do the same again tomorrow.

The most underrated feature of a house is storage. If you don't have any, get some—it's the only way for things to have a place. Some say you can never be too rich or too thin, but I say you can never have too much storage space! In an organised house which has a place for everything and minimal clutter, incidental tidying is much easier, and it stays tidy for longer with less effort. If you have time before baby is born, have a good spring clean and sort out the house from top to bottom. If you already have little ones, put aside some time when there's an extra pair of hands around, like on holidays or weekends.

Avoid stockpiling things you don't really use or need—old magazines, and outgrown or damaged toys or books. Give them to a friend or charity, hold a garage sale or sell them on the internet.

Sort out wardrobes and pack away clothes that are out of season, worn only on special occasions or currently the wrong size (for maternity or children). I do this and the best part is that it forces me to sort out my wardrobe twice a year, which would otherwise only happen when I move house. It is the ideal opportunity to minimise. Only keep items in your wardrobe which fit you well and which you actually wear.

Getting your surroundings really organised will make you feel lighter, more energised and more in control as you tackle your new life head-on.

TIDY TOYS

Forget the 'terrible twos' . . . the bane of my existence is the terrible toys! A house with young children can easily look like a preschool explosion (my house). It's not worth cleaning up all the toys at lunchtime or nap time, as you end up putting away the same stuff at dinnertime and again at bedtime. Yes, the mess you trip over can drive you crazy, but all you can really do is be sorted and have a place for everything. After that, don't stress about the mess all day, as it will return to haunt you. Focus on something else that really needs to be done.

Also, make sure to teach any child old enough to follow simple instructions (i.e. from about one year old) to pack up things after they play and to help with the big tidy-up before bedtime. It has to be routine, it can be fun and the effort is well worth it. They are forming habits with their surroundings and belongings, whether you are instructing them or not. So teach them good habits early on, otherwise you're looking at 20 years of nagging and picking up after someone!

Another tactic is toy rotation. All toys do not need to be accessible at all times. Young children lose interest in toys quickly and will pull out everything they can reach in the course of a day, leaving a total disaster. Absence makes the toddler heart grow fonder of toys that have been out of sight and hence out of mind. Having toys stored away is also handy on quiet days, rainy days, sick days or mummy's-having-a-lie-down-today days. Try not to let toddlers have access to anything with 1001 pieces, otherwise there'll be pieces in your shoe, in the toilet, in the bin, in the freezer, under the rug, throughout the sandpit, in the washing machine and under your pillow.

Check if there's a toy library in your area. These are great for children who get bored easily. You pay a toy hire fee, but it's nothing compared to buying new toys which they're tired of in two days. Alternatively, swap toys, books and videos with friends to keep them engaged. I've passed around everything from pop-up cubby houses to the playhouse kitchen sink with my friends.

Housework

There is no avoiding it. It has always been; it will always be. Even if you work outside the home or are fortunate enough to have hired help in this department, there are still many endless everyday tasks. Be realistic about the state of your house when inhabited by small children and let less important things occasionally slide.

In really busy times, take some shortcuts and save your sanity. Really, what does it matter if you don't put away the clean washing for four days and take things from the pile to wear? (That's my story and I'm sticking to it.) Save the 'perfect house' presentation for entertaining on a special occasion or trying to sell a house, but otherwise being organised and consistent will keep your surroundings clean and tidy enough to ensure a balanced lifestyle. If you stop sweating the small stuff, you'll most likely do a better job with you and your family, and that's what really counts—people.

IRONING

I truly hate this one. Do you really need to iron absolutely everything infants wear? If you get to the clothes soon after they are dry and fold them well, they remain surprisingly flat and wrinkle free. And even if you put a child of this age in a clean and perfectly pressed outfit, there are several things which happen between dressing the child and getting out the door: dribbling, regurgitating, snacking, crawling, wrestling, snotty-nose wiping, and smudging with crayons or toothpaste.

Go for easy-care clothes where possible. For example, T-shirt and board-short type fabrics wash well, dry quickly and rarely need pressing. Little woven cotton shirts with tiny button-down collars and pleated linen party dresses are gorgeous, but should be saved for special occasions unless you happen to really enjoy ironing or have someone else do it for you.

Finding extra time

A great way to find extra time is to trade childcare with a friend in the same situation. This gets easier as your children get older, so if you don't already have friends nearby in the same situation, foster those mothers group or preschool relationships. By the time you're busy with baby number two, you'll have friends you trust to look after your toddler and even the baby on occasion. Active toddlers really enjoy playing at a little friend's house with all their toys and you know your children will be in a safe, child-friendly environment.

Babysitting swaps are also good for nighttime babysitting so you and your partner can get out on a date. It works well for all involved. Someone gets a night out, with a babysitter they trust. And the babysitting mum gets a night away from her environment, where she would probably be doing something like laundry. But at someone else's house, so long as the little ones sleep, you can relax on the sofa and watch a movie or nap. And get your own night out with free babysitting next time!

STEP 3: SCHEDULE FOR SUCCESS

Create a weekly schedule using your list of priorities. Start by adding the known items such as meal times, school times and scheduled activities, then slot in the more flexible items around them. I have included one of mine with a basic framework as an example (see Table 3.1). I keep a separate 'to do' list of chores handy, as they quickly clutter the weekly schedule. I put the time slot in for 'to do' items, then consult the job list when the time comes. It sounds like a bore, but everyone's life involves things which have to be done like completing paperwork for school, paying bills, filing bank statements and finding all the pieces of the puzzles in the bottom of the toy boxes. These are not pressing items, but they hang over your head and it's really satisfying to actually cross things off the list.

Be specific and lock items in; if it's not on the schedule, it won't happen. Find pairs or groups of jobs which can be done together, alternated or rotated. For example, if you want to change the bed linen twice a month and can go two weeks between bathroom cleanings, then alternate between these two in the same time slot on your schedule. Right now you may start each week with the same list of chores you started

TABLE 3.1 My schedule as a writer with young children

	MONDAY	TUESDAY	WEDNESDAY	THURSDAY	FRIDAY	SATURDAY	SUNDAY
7.00	Breakfast	Breakfast	Breakfast	Breakfast	Breakfast	Breakfast	Breakfast
8.45	Preschool	Preschool				Exercise	
9.30	Groceries	Mothers group	Kindy-gym 45 min				
10.00	Freezer cooking	(Shop/cook alternative)	Play at park				
11.30					Swimming		
12.00	Lunch	Lunch	Lunch	Lunch	Lunch	Lunch	Lunch
1.00	Nap (kids)	Write	Nap	Nap	Nap/Write?	Nap/Write?	Nap/Write?
2.30	Preschool	Preschool	(Run w/kids b4 dinner?)	(Run w/kids b4 dinner?)			(Shop/cook alternative)
5.00	Dinner	Dinner	Dinner	Dinner	Dinner	Dinner	Dinner
6.30			Kung-fu (Ben)	(Run w/kids after dinner?)			
7.30	Dance (2 hrs)	Write	Write	Write			
8.30				Write?	Movie		

with last week. Once you break up the work and schedule it in, it's much easier to keep up and even find more free time when you don't feel you *should* be cleaning or sorting. Remember, this is a strategy to make life easier, *not* an attempt at domestic perfection.

When creating your weekly schedule, put in jobs for children too. They can tidy their toys, make their beds, put away their clothes, and help with food preparation and setting the table from a young age. The sooner you give them responsibility, the faster they'll gain confidence in their own abilities and also learn you are not their slave!

Your schedule may live on a whiteboard or pin-board in the kitchen or family area so other family members can follow it. I keep mine on my computer desktop for easy modification from month to month. Remember it's a framework, a guide to help you prioritise and use time efficiently, but all is negotiable and flexible. If baby is sick or you're having a particularly bad day, forget the schedule, forget the house, get someone to bring you takeaway for dinner and do what you need to do—take care of the people first.

Juggling the essentials of sleeping, eating well, exercising and being a mum seems easier when it's mapped out on a timetable and you can see it all fits. The amount of detail you include is up to you. I believe everyone can use a version of this to get organised. Just as running a good business requires a plan, so too does a busy life.

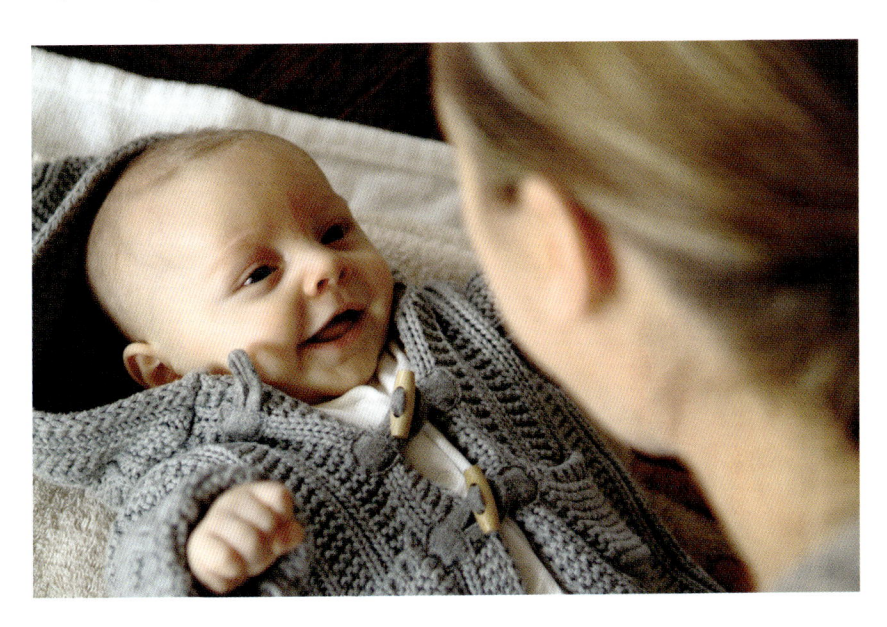

Action

Recruit extra hands and sort toys, clothes, kitchen cupboards and anywhere else bursting at the seams

Focus on what's really important and forget ideals of perfection for things that don't matter in the big picture

Collect favourite meal ideas or recipes

Make a list of what you do each week, and what you'd like to add

Get a whiteboard, chalkboard or poster, make a schedule, put it somewhere visible

Delegate jobs to partners and children as appropriate

STEP 4: START NOW

Your plans now look great, on paper. All you have to do is start, right now. Not after that party coming up, not next Monday—today, right now. Everything you do from this moment on can be geared towards great health for you and your family if you choose. Make the commitment. Procrastinating will only make tasks seem bigger than they are and set you back further.

Try your timetable and modify it as necessary. Give it a few weeks to see if you have been realistic about how much you do and when you do it. Make changes, but remember not to sacrifice things you decided are important, and use all the time-saving shortcuts you can. Once applied to the real world, your plan must remain dynamic to survive. You have to cut yourself a little slack and not feel pressured to perform as a perfectly regimented soldier at all times. Remember, it's just a way to help you stay on track—not a tactic to add more pressure!

The point in having a plan is so you know what's coming up and can be prepared. For example, if you have exercise scheduled for the day, get your shoes, music or DVD ready to go. Keep the walking pram out, packed with a water bottle, a spare nappy and wipes, a baby blanket and hats ready to go when the time comes. And two minutes stolen here and there doing a simple exercise can give you a full-body workout by the end of the day, without you really noticing the time it took. If things don't go to plan, reschedule what you missed. Don't tell yourself it's too hard and you can't do it all; ask when you will do it.

From now on, make Yoda's words your mantra: 'Do not try. Do.'

PART 11
Energy to burn

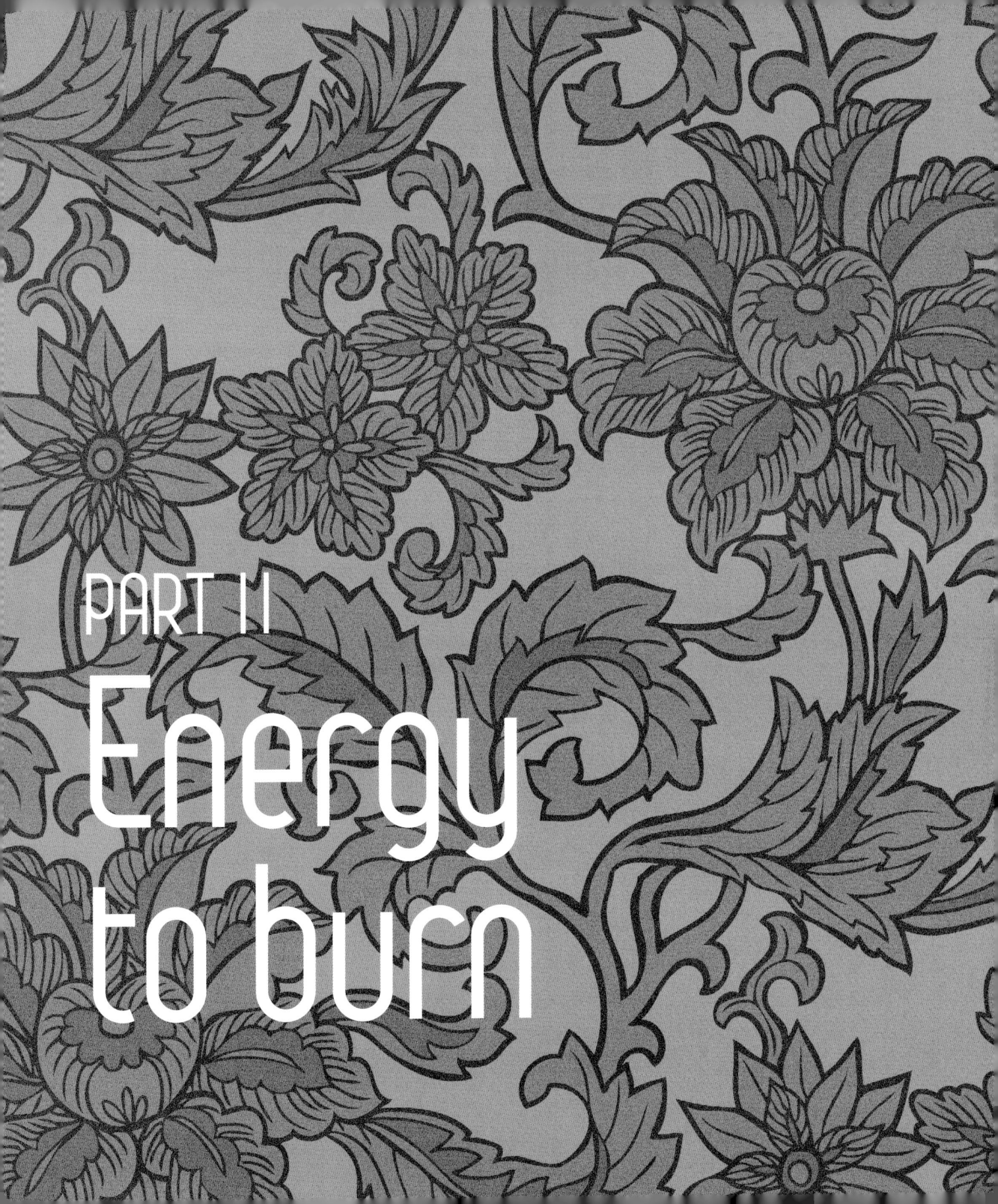

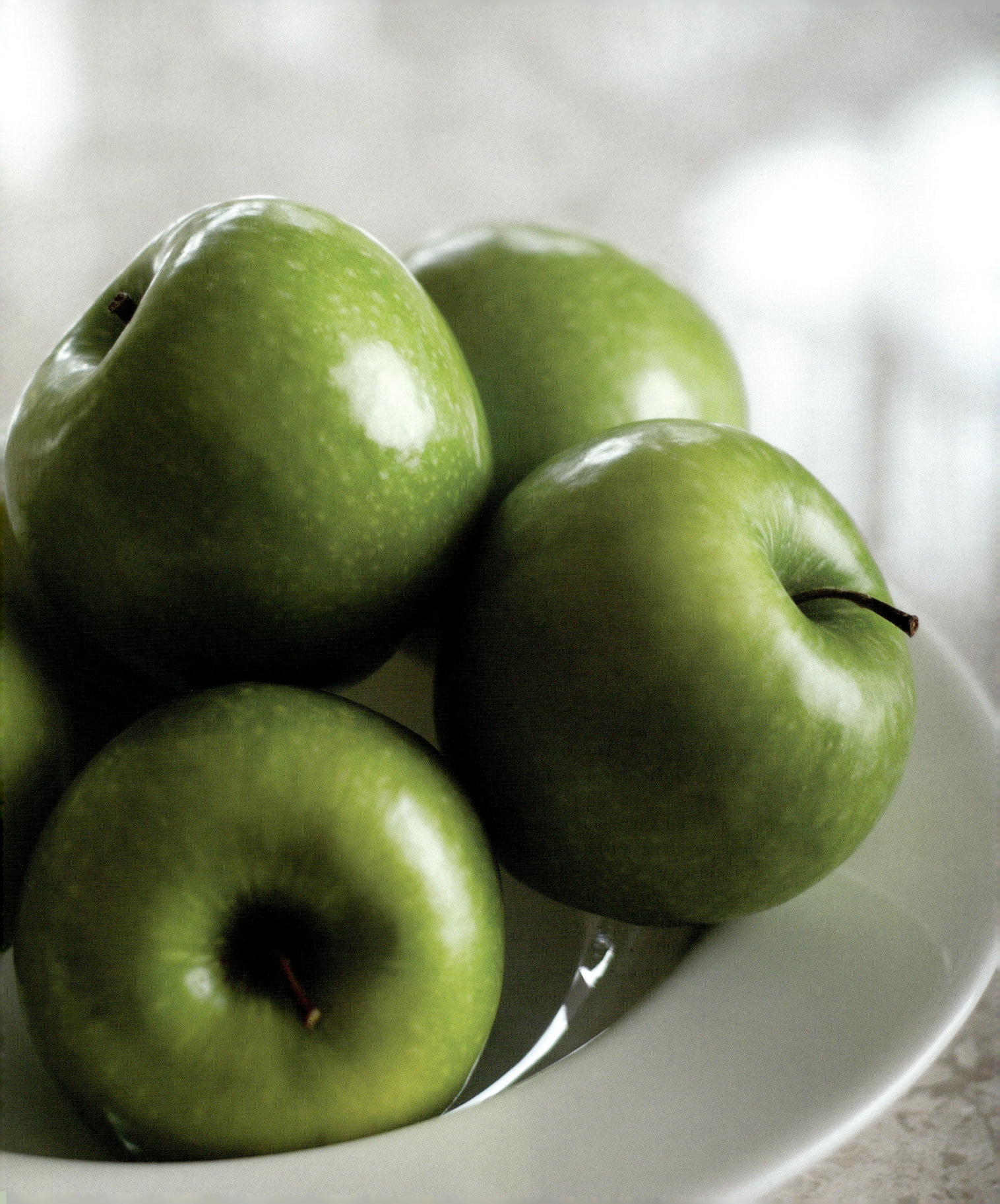

Energy balance and metabolism: Don't fight the system

Ready?
Brush up on how your body works

Dieting ruins your metabolism

Learn how to muscle out fat

All the facts on fat, carbohydrate, protein and alcohol

Weight-loss tips that work with your body, not against it

Nutrition and exercise are serious scientific fields, but the simple physiological facts of nutrition and exercise we are taught in school and by public health organisations such as the National Heart Foundation and the National Health and Medical Research Council are accurate, practical and backed by research. Yet unscrupulous parties in the diet and fitness industry are forever on the prowl, trying to get a finger in the purses of the unsuspecting and the eternally hopeful.

DIET IS A FOUR-LETTER WORD

My number-one rule for all fit and fabulous mums is: don't diet!

Diets simply do not work. Studies show most people who go on a diet regain all the weight they lose, and often more. Everyone knows diets don't work, so why is there a hopeful sucker born every minute? Otherwise extremely intelligent women I know discuss the hot new diets they're on from one season to the next; I'm stunned they just can't accept the scientific truth about how nutrition works in our bodies and that everything else is just hype.

Diet fads and useless products usually start with one scientific fact as a basis, so it sounds plausible. Manufacturers peddle subscriptions to products that are not only pure marketing hype, but will do more harm than good when you have to eat real food again one day. Results claimed to be achieved or actually achieved by these manufactured supplements, powders, shakes, pills or bars can be reached and sustained more effectively, safely and less expensively with normal, natural foods and regular exercise. Everyone knows this.

Those of you accustomed to dieting are probably panicking and wondering how on earth to move the baby bulge without going on a severe diet. Don't worry, we'll get into proper nutrition and positive eating in the next few chapters; positive eating is the opposite of dieting (what *to* eat, rather than what *not* to eat) because to live, you have to eat.

There's a lot of attitude, philosophy and psychology tied up in how and what you eat and for most people on a diet the problem is not their body, it's their head! Remember, the facts of metabolism, exercise and nutrition don't go far without addressing such issues as stress, priorities, time management, habits, attitude, goals, motivation and lifestyle.

The scientific community knows a lot about metabolism and exercise physiology. It is an area of increasing proven knowledge. When I read the hot diet fads that come out every spring, I instantly know why they will fail. Not because I'm pessimistic, but because I know how the human body works—and how it doesn't!

Be a scientist; question everything. If it sounds too good to be true, it probably is. This chapter explains what you *really* need to know about getting in shape, so you'll have the confidence to make the best health choices for you. My hope is that with the correct physiological information about how your body uses and stores fuel, you'll never consider a diet pill, supplement or quick-fix diet again. Ever.

WHAT IS METABOLISM?

You've most likely heard of the term metabolism in reference to the many weight-loss diets, pills and potions on the market. Metabolism comes down to just one basic mathematical equation,

'There's no easy way. If there were, I would have bought it. And believe me, it would be one of my favourite things!'

Oprah Winfrey (on weight loss),
O Magazine, February 2005

which you don't even need to calculate precisely so long as you understand how it works.

The term 'energy' refers to the fuel (kilojoules) your body uses all the time—to exercise, rest, breathe, pump blood, sleep, repair, grow, and build babies. Energy demands vary depending on what you're doing, but if the car's running, even if it's just idling, it requires fuel. 'Metabolic rate' or 'metabolism' refers to the amount of energy you're using at any given time, or how far down your foot is on the accelerator, if you like. Sleep is like idling in that it requires very little energy, but you still breathe, your heart beats, your blood flows, you may be digesting, or repairing or growing tissues. During sleep or rest, your metabolic rate (or metabolism) is near its lowest and is called your resting metabolic rate (RMR). Even lower than your RMR is your basal metabolic rate (BMR) which is usually only used for clinical purposes and is calculated by measuring energy use just after waking, 12–18 hours after a meal, in a temperature-controlled environment. This is the energy you need to stay alive. On top of your basal metabolic rate, the body uses energy throughout the day for digesting and absorbing food, regulating body temperature, and for physical activity. Hormones, infection or illness, and drugs can also alter metabolic rate. Once you get out of bed, your metabolic rate accelerates to keep up with the increasing demand for energy required to move your body. When you exercise, your metabolic rate rises even more, and slows again later as you relax with a book.

The idea that our metabolism adjusts to maintain stable body weight in the short term is called the 'set point theory'. If you suddenly and drastically reduce your energy intake, your metabolism slows to fight the weight loss by as much as 15–20 per cent! Conversely, if you eat more than usual, your metabolism speeds up (in the short term) to process the extra fuel. This explains why it is hard to sustain weight loss achieved by severe short-term diets. The set point can change slowly over time through a sustained energy excess or deficiency. So, to lose weight and keep it off, a slower, gradual loss will allow your metabolism to adjust accordingly and readjust the set point.

Metabolism during pregnancy and breastfeeding

After pregnancy, even though you may have stored extra fat, your metabolic rate is most likely higher than before pregnancy as your body has become a factory—a manufacturing plant for making, protecting and nourishing baby. The flurry of activity in growing a placenta, producing hormones, building a baby or two and producing milk all uses lots of energy. Even if you weren't active during pregnancy and lost fitness and muscle mass, your body still works hard to support two people, especially while breastfeeding. This is a *great* time to start exercising, increasing your lean body tissue and metabolism.

Breastfeeding requires lots of nutritious energy, so it's important not to go on very restrictive diets during this time. But you can start losing baby weight right away. In fact it's easier than if you're not breastfeeding—add exercise and you'll start using that stored fat. Occasionally, women producing a lot of milk may need to cut back on exercise to sustain feeding if they're losing weight too quickly.

Sometimes it's hard to lose *all* baby fat until after feeding stops as your body keeps some in reserve for milk production. But don't stress about losing every inch right away. You can still attend that party with a new mum's two best accessories guaranteed to grab attention from all: a gorgeous new baby and a fabulous cleavage!

KILOJOULES AND FUEL

When it comes to fuelling the human body, the car analogy is most effective. You'd only put three things in a car to ensure it runs well: fuel, water and oil. The fuel is for energy, the water for cooling and the oil to lubricate. In the same way, there are only three things your body really needs:
- food for energy, building and repair
- water for tasks like cooling and transport
- vitamins and minerals—like the oil in the car, they keep things running smoothly.

Kilojoules (kJ) and kilocalories (Kcal) are both common units to measure the energy derived from food. They are just different systems adopted in different parts of the world to measure exactly the same thing. The scientific definition of one calorie is the amount of heat energy required to raise the temperature of one gram of water by one degree Celsius. One thousand calories equals one kilocalorie (Kcal) and Kcals are common unit used on food labels (which most people abbreviate to say 'calories').

Kilojoules are the System International (SI) form of measuring heat energy. One kilocalorie equals 4.186 kilojoules. But don't get bogged down in the numbers and conversions. When reading food labels, it is more important to examine *total grams* of types of fuel and the percentages.

The fuel or energy we eat, store and use comes from food—specifically carbohydrates, protein and fat. Each of these fuel sources contains different amounts of kilojoules per gram, with fat being the most energy dense. The section on fuel sources later in this chapter explains this in more detail.

Metabolic rate determines how much of the energy you eat is used or 'burned', and how much you store—and there are many factors influencing this. Metabolism is just a piece of the puzzle and cannot be blamed for everything. Genetics determine your body type and frame—whether you're tall or short, and have a large or petite skeletal frame. But on top of that, environmental factors such as diet and exercise determine how efficiently your body burns fuel and also your body shape.

BODY COMPOSITION

Body composition refers to the ratio of fat to lean body mass (muscle, bone, organs etc.), usually as the percentage of the body made up of fat. For example, an endurance athlete may be very lean and have 11 per cent body fat, while an overweight 'armchair' athlete may have 36 per cent body fat. If the latter weighs 100 kg, he has 36 kg of fat to lug around. In fact, if you put on more fat weight, your body has to grow more muscle to carry it, so you gain even more total weight.

There are several methods to measure or estimate body composition, and these differ greatly in complexity and accuracy. You'll find tests and devices for this purpose in fitness centres, elite sports training facilities, clinical health and rehabilitation centres and department stores and on television shopping channels. Look, you really *do not* need to know your exact percentage of body fat. It's just a number. You know if you have extra kilos to lose—you know if it's squishy or bulging where it used to be firm and flat. Some gym junkies or bodybuilders get obsessed by this number, much like golfers and their handicaps, but when you've got babies, details like this just don't matter. The easiest measure of getting back into shape is how well your clothes fit.

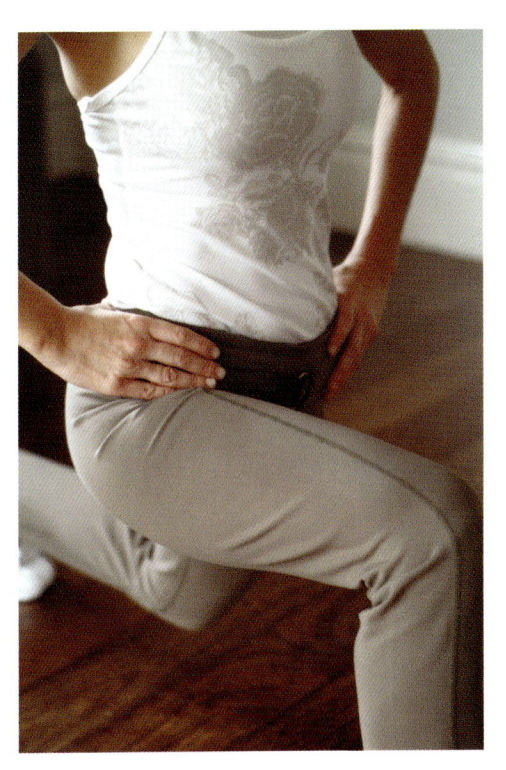

TABLE 4.1
BMI classification of weight in adults 19–35 years

Underweight	<18.5
Normal range	18.5–24.9
Overweight	>25
Pre-obese	25–29.9
Obese class I	30–34.9
Obese class II	35–39.9
Obese class III	40

(www.heartfoundation.com.au)

Even the scales can lie. Muscle is a heavier, denser tissue than fat. With every gram of carbohydrate we store in our muscles for energy, we also need to store nearly three grams of water. So muscle is a very hydrated tissue. What does this mean, really?

Well, compare two women: Sally is 165 cm tall; so is Jane as they are identical twins and have exactly the same skeletal frame. Sally jogs, lifts weights, does yoga, is training for a half-marathon and eats a balanced diet. She wears a size 10 and her body looks fit; her tummy is flat, her waist is smaller than her hips and chest, she has some muscle definition and is quite lean. Jane, however, does little deliberate physical activity and eats a lot of takeaway and fatty snacks. She wears a size 12–14 because of extra padding all over. Her tummy is about the same girth as her chest and her hips are larger. She is obviously carrying considerably more fat than her sister. This is not extreme; Jane is not obese. But the interesting thing is that both women weigh the same. Jane is lugging around extra volume in the form of lots of spongy fat tissue, while Sally is packed with dense, tight, heavier muscle.

Body composition is measured in elite sports clinics with the 'gold standard' test of underwater weighing (hydrostatic weighing). In less formal fitness settings, more variable—that is, less reliable—methods are used, such as bioelectrical impedance analysis and skinfold calipers. One common method for estimating body composition is with a simple calculation called the body mass index (BMI): weight in kilograms ÷ height in metres squared. So, for a person weighing 63 kg who is 165 cm tall, their BMI would be calculated as: 63 kg ÷ 1.65 m^2 = 23.14.

It is important to note that this does not directly measure fat percentage. The numbers reflect the relationship between how heavy you are for your height and hence the likelihood that you are overweight.

BMI is useful as a guide to general health and the recommendations vary for different age groups. Table 4.1 is for men and women aged 19–35 years. A BMI of 19–25 is considered healthy for adults of this age, but for those over 35 years the normal range is 21–27.

The main problem with BMI is that it does not account for body frame or muscle mass. For example, most professional rugby players would be classified as obese because they are heavy for their height as they have a lot of muscle—yet they are lean and very fit. This is not usually an issue for an average woman after a baby, but it is important to recognise the possible inaccuracies and treat the results as a guide only.

THE EFFECT OF BODY COMPOSITION ON METABOLISM

Body composition affects metabolism, weight loss and energy levels. Muscle, being a dense, heavy tissue, is very 'expensive' to maintain in terms of kilojoules used, compared to fat. Muscles need lots of nutrients, water and energy to repair, build and move your body.

Back to Sally and Jane. This all means Sally is a fast-burning machine. When she sits next to Jane to watch a movie, Sally is burning more fuel than Jane, who has a sluggish metabolism. When they climb stairs, Sally burns more fuel than Jane. Even though they carry the same total weight around, since Sally's engine revs higher—having a higher metabolic rate as a starting point—she burns more fuel in everything she does, just like a V8 engine burns through petrol.

If they both eat a pizza, Jane will store more of the energy, but Sally will burn it off faster. A fast-burning machine uses fuel more efficiently, stores less, uses stored energy more easily, has better endurance and feels energetic.

So, how do you become a fast-burning machine?

You train for it. You alter your body composition for relatively more muscle and less fat. Don't be afraid of 'bulking up'—it's very difficult for women to get big, bulging muscles, even if you train specifically for it. Chapter 7 looks at exercise in detail, but for now I'll just assure you that resistance training is the secret weapon for getting in the best shape ever. With the right nutrition, it can transform a soft, sluggish marshmallow into a trim, energetic fast-burning machine.

THE ENERGY EQUATION

Every theory ever touted regarding diet, exercise and weight loss comes down to this basic mathematical equation:

energy in = energy out   **weight is maintained, no change**
energy in > (is greater than) energy out   **weight gain (energy surplus)**
energy in < (is less than) energy out   **weight loss (energy deficit)**

If you use the same amount of kilojoules you consume, you maintain body weight. If you eat more than you use, you store it and gain weight. If you use more energy than you eat, you lose weight by using stored energy as well.

> 'Quit now, you'll never make it. If you disregard this advice, you'll be halfway there?'
>
> David Zucker

It *is* as simple as that.

Obsession with the kilojoules you eat is only relevant if you know how many you're expending. Kilojoule intake on its own does not determine whether or not you lose weight. A diet plan may tell you to consume only a set number of kilojoules a day—but without individual information on your resting metabolic rate (related to your body composition) and how much incidental activity and exercise you do, there is no way to universally declare everyone will lose weight on this prescribed amount. If it happens to be less energy than you usually eat, you will most likely lose weight initially. But when you stop the diet, as your body has become more competent at preserving fuel stores (and your metabolic rate drops), you easily put the weight back on, usually with some extra for your trouble.

This describes classic 'yo-yo' dieting and shows that although food intake greatly influences your weight, exercise is essential to increase the 'energy out' and tip the equation in your favour. Trying to lose weight without exercise means your 'energy in' has to be too restrictive to maintain in the long term, and the adverse effects on your metabolism work against you. Your body literally goes into 'self-preservation' mode and rations stored energy to get through the 'famine'. This is handy should you be stranded on a desert island without food, but not great for losing a few kilos of extra baby weight. As exercise increases your metabolism, it can help the equation work in your favour, even without significantly reducing food intake.

ENERGY BALANCE AND METABOLISM 53

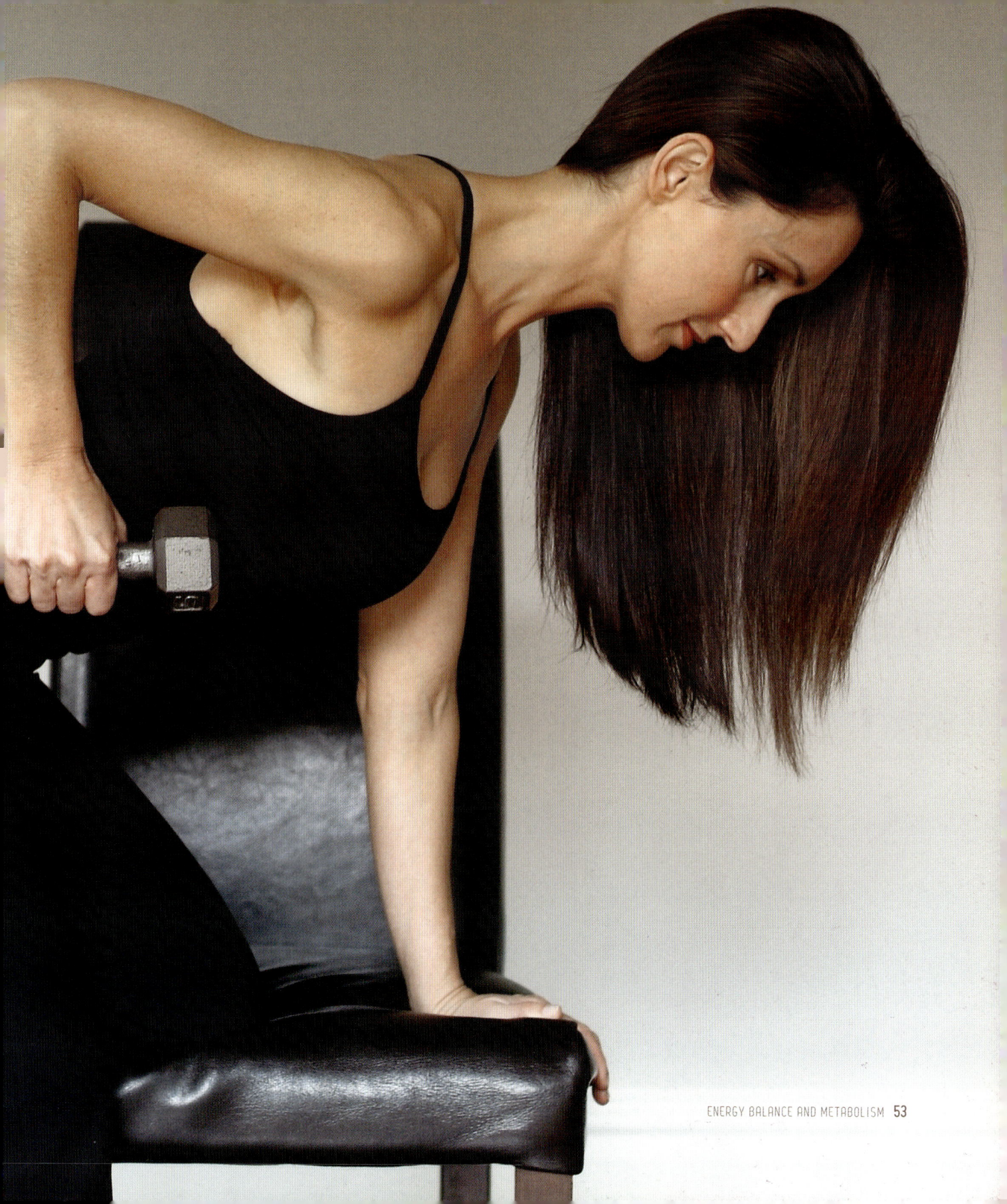

Becoming a good loser

If you try a very restrictive diet to lose weight, you cannot control the type of weight lost. There is no way to tell your body to use up the fat and keep the lean tissue. And unfortunately, female bodies of child-bearing age often hang onto fat in case it's needed for insulation, protection and reproduction. Very low energy regimes—such as soup diets, meal-replacement drinks and bars—produce short-lived, misleading results. They can seem to melt the kilos at first, but this is mostly a decrease in muscle tissue and its stored carbohydrate and water—so you may not necessarily have lost much fat. Severe diets ruin your metabolism as they tell your body to store energy (not use it) because you lose muscle.

Body circumference measurements often indicate fat loss better than weighing on scales. Measurements taken each month, at various locations such as the waist, chest, upper arms and thighs, are an easy way to monitor your body's response to lifestyle changes you make. And this gives more information about the type of weight you're losing. Because fat is a less dense, more spongy tissue, a kilogram of fat is much larger in volume than a kilogram of muscle. It's like comparing a kilo of scotch fillet with a kilo of popcorn, to exaggerate the point. If you're carrying a lot of popcorn, it would be hard to notice if you drop a steak or two from underneath it. But if you dropped kilograms of popcorn from the outside, your circumference measurements would definitely show the loss, and so would your clothes size.

The key to effective long-term fat loss is exercise. You can lose weight over time if you just restrict energy intake (that is, diet), but you can't tell your body what *type* of weight to lose if you diet. But exercise can.

Exercise stimulates the body to preserve and build lean muscle tissue to store water and carbohydrate for fuel. So, it uses stored fat to meet energy demands above the amount you have eaten.

You just need a balanced diet—chapter 5 details this—which, when plugged into the energy equation along with your exercise, leaves you short of fuel for the week (in other words, the energy you've taken in is less than the energy you've expended). And this is exactly what you want—to lose weight while maintaining or increasing your metabolism.

FUEL SOURCES

There are three essential nutrients used as energy by the human body: carbohydrate, fat and protein. Alcohol also provides energy (kilojoules), but is far from being an essential nutrient.

Fat

Fat is a very sneaky nutrient. It hides in things like plain biscuits and salad dressings and holds on tight once it gets into the body. It can easily add 'empty' kilojoules to your intake which, if you don't use them, you store and gain weight.

Fat is very dense in kilojoules compared to the other fuel sources. Fat contains about 38 kJ (9 Kcal) for every gram, which is more than twice as much energy as protein or carbohydrate. Most foods and meals contain a combination of the three types of fuel, and all good weight-loss advice encourages choosing foods with lower proportions of fat, so you can lower your kilojoule intake and tip the energy balance equation more in your favour.

Not all fats are equal. In terms of *energy* they are, but not in terms of health. All sources of fat contain a mix of different types of fats described in terms of 'saturation'. This term refers to the chemical structure of the fat molecule (how saturated or 'packed' it is with hydrogen atoms). **Saturated fat** is the baddie and is found in animal products and coconut and palm oils. It is usually solid at room temperature, like butter or lard. These fats are nasty because they increase 'bad' cholesterol in the body and fatty deposits sticking to the walls of blood vessels, and contribute to cardiovascular disease, now the biggest killer of women in Australia. Cardiovascular disease is the term used to describe heart and blood vessel diseases, which currently kill one in three Australians by heart attack or stroke. That's how real lifestyle diseases are. And they have become environmentally hereditary—we are passing these diseases on to our children, not with genes, but with our habits.

Then there are the **unsaturated fats**, which are usually liquid at room temperature. Oils high in monounsaturated fat such as olive, peanut and canola oils are healthier substitutes for saturated fats like butter. Vegetable, nut and seed oils high in polyunsaturated fats like sunflower, soy, flaxseed and canola (again) are also sources of essential fats called omega-6 fatty acids. Omega-3 fats, from fish such as salmon, tuna, sardines and trout, are important to prevent blood clotting, lowering the risk of stroke and cardiovascular disease. We need small amounts of omega-6 and omega-3 essential fatty acids as they are necessary for producing hormones, for brain development, vision, growth and immunity.

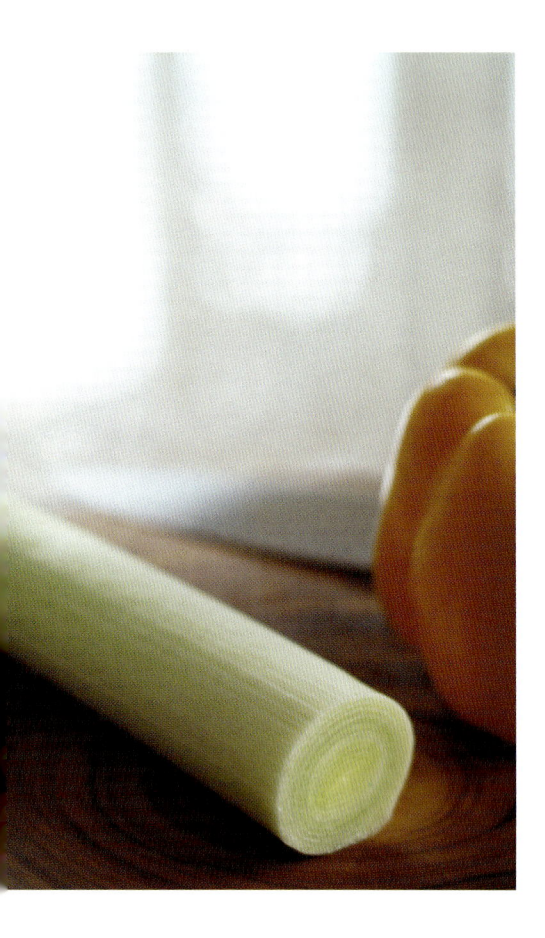

Trans fats are probably the worst fats of all. They are manufactured fats found in deep-fried food and some processed foods such as some margarines and biscuits. They are usually labelled as 'hydrogenated' or 'partially hydrogenated oils'. Basically, trans fats are made when hydrogen gas is bubbled through unsaturated oil, 'saturating' it and making it solid at room temperature. Trans fats may be even worse for heart health than saturated fats, so read the food labels and steer clear.

Although some fats are referred to as 'good' and 'essential', this is not a cue to actively increase your total fat consumption. It is a guide for *which* fats to choose in your diet, as we do need some fat. Remember that it is unlikely you are deficient in essential fats and that all fats are equal in terms of kilojoules. So eating lots of 'good' fats won't help at all with the energy equation, or losing weight. More fat of any kind is still more kilojoules to work off or store!

What you do with this information is choose foods with the *right* kind of fats—olive oil instead of butter; fish over fatty red meat. Reading food labels is essential to monitor how much and what type of fat you're consuming—but preferably most food you eat should not be labelled or processed at all! The National Health and Medical Research Council recommends that for weight maintenance no more than 30 per cent of daily energy should come from fat, and no more than 10 per cent total cholesterol. For weight loss, the total fat can be dropped to 20 per cent.

After fat is eaten and digested, it is absorbed into the bloodstream. Then, if it is not used, it travels to storage—mostly in adipose tissue and some in muscles. Adipose tissue is the term for stored fat deposits all over the body—on the stomach, thighs, bottom, breasts, arms, legs, under the skin and in between organs—you name it, it sticks there!

We are very efficient at absorbing digested fat and we do not excrete the excess. The human body has an unlimited capacity to store fat. If fat cells fill up, and you continue to eat more fat and don't use the energy, the body just makes more fat cells to store it. When fat is required as an energy source, the fat in the bloodstream and muscles is used first, and the fat in adipose tissue last.

Eating *some* fat is beneficial even when trying to lose weight. A total 'fat ban', such as in very low-energy diets, teaches the body to store fat more readily and hold onto it tighter. Fat also enhances the palatability of food, making it juicier, more flavourful and hence more satisfying. For example, just a drop of sesame oil is wonderfully fragrant in a stir-fry. A tiny drizzle of hazelnut oil with balsamic vinegar on mixed salad leaves adds a delectable flavour. If you love chocolate with your coffee as I do, have a little—without it, I'd eat three plain biscuits and still want the chocolate! The more satisfying the meal, the less you eat and the longer before you're hungry again, so you eat less total kilojoules during the day. Trying for a no-fat diet leaves you feeling deprived and most likely overeating to feel satisfied, which can result in a higher kilojoule intake than if you ate a little fat in the first place!

Here's another tip: **if you crave some fat, eat it at breakfast** when you have the day to use the energy—not at dinner when you have the night to store it.

Overall, if you're trying to lose weight, this is the nutrient to reduce. If you substitute fat with protein or carbohydrate you'll instantly halve kilojoules without starving yourself.

Carbohydrate

Carbohydrate has been a controversial fuel in recent years, but mainly in the popular media. Health professionals have known how carbohydrates work for a long time, and that knowledge has not significantly changed.

Carbohydrates are not *bad*, they are not fattening, and they cannot easily turn into fat. The only connection they have with gaining fat is indirect. Carbohydrates are the preferred fuel source in the body, so if you overeat carbohydrates, you will have a constant supply of energy to use and so will store more fat eaten.

Carbohydrates can only be turned into fat as an absolute last resort in cases of extreme carbohydrate overfeeding. It is not a simple process; they have to be broken down and rebuilt into fat if the body absolutely has nowhere else for them to go. It is a very inefficient process—it costs about a quarter of the energy just to do it—and so we never convert a significant quantity. The excessive volume of total food which has to be consumed to do this at all is much more disturbing, and thankfully extremely rare. But once someone says the body is able to do it, people assume the body *does* do it, hence the 'low-carb' diet craze.

If you eat proportionately less carbohydrate then you will eat more protein and more fat—more bacon, for example, a favourite of some low-carb diets. But the easiest thing to store as fat is FAT! So why would you be more concerned about carbohydrate turning into fat than eating fat itself? A diet high in protein and animal fats (which often go together) is linked to increased bowel cancer, particularly in diets that are also low in fibre. Fruits and vegetables, which are high in carbohydrates, also provide many important vitamins and minerals, so it's vital not to cut down on these. The message gets very convoluted when someone turns a grain of truth into a hot new diet. Biochemical details often don't add up to much in real-world application, so stick with the big picture.

The other interesting fact about energy use in the human body is that 'fat burns in a carbohydrate flame'. This means you actually *need* carbohydrate for the physiological process that uses the fat you eat and stored body fat—you cannot get rid of fat without carbs! So that just punches another hole in the low-carb craze.

Carbohydrates in the body are found in muscle tissue, the liver and the bloodstream where they are transported to muscles needing energy for movement. They are an essential, most readily accessed form of energy. They contain about 17 kJ (4 Kcal) per gram. Like the fuel tank in a car, the liver and muscles store carbohydrates, and once these are used and depleted they must be replaced at the next meal.

Carbohydrate is the body's preferred source of energy and fat is the reserve tank. You do use a mix of both all the time, but this is controlled by the amount of carbohydrate available. If you eat too large a volume of carbohydrates, or of any fuel, you will have so much energy readily available that you'll never be able to deplete it and never start using any stored fat. But the real problem here is too much *total energy*. It's the energy equation again: too much in and not enough out.

Just like fats, although all carbohydrates have the same amount of kilojoules, they are not all equal in terms of health and function in the body. Carbohydrates are often described as 'simple' or 'complex' due to their chemical structure, although the terms 'sugars' and 'starches' are more accurate.

Sugars or simple carbohydrates are generally sweet. Examples of foods high in simple sugars are jelly beans (glucose), fruit juice (fructose), milk sugar (lactose), table sugar (sucrose), honey and maple syrup. Like sneaky fats, they are often packed into processed foods such as breakfast cereals and sweet biscuits. They are easy to eat in large quantities, providing too many kilojoules without a 'full' feeling. One of the worst offenders is high-fructose corn syrup, manufactured by adding fructose to the natural glucose in corn. Many people see the word 'corn' and think it can't be too unhealthy, but they don't realise high-fructose corn syrup is a sugar with whopping amounts of kilojoules. It is a cheaper and sweeter alternative to sugar and is used in many processed foods, from soft drinks and juices to yoghurts and biscuits. It is also found in many foods marketed to children. It trains their tastebuds to crave sweeter and sweeter foods and is accused of contributing to increasing obesity.

As sugars are digested and absorbed quickly into the bloodstream, they do not provide *sustained* energy. Our blood sugar (glucose) is very carefully regulated. If blood glucose rises quickly, our body controls this by releasing lots of insulin to remove it to storage. Energy more slowly absorbed gives a constant stream of readily available fuel.

Complex carbohydrates contain starch and fibre. Starches provide a great source of energy, and because they are slower to break down than simple sugars, they make you feel fuller and have more energy for longer. Once digested, if not needed immediately, starch energy is stored in the muscles and liver as glycogen. Examples of foods high in starches are cereals, vegetables, fruit, rice, pasta and bread. Starches also contain fibre, a non-digestible plant material like cellulose, pectin and gum. Fibre passes through our digestive system and plays very important roles in 'sweeping out' the pipes, helping prevent bowel cancer and lowering cholesteral. Whole grains and cereals, beans, corn, pumpkin and seeds are all good sources of fibre.

In terms of choosing the best carbohydrates, starches win over sugars because:
- you feel fuller after eating them; they delay hunger and help control appetite
- they are more slowly absorbed, providing longer-lasting energy and keeping blood sugar levels more stable
- they also contain fibre and often more vitamins and minerals than sugars, which are essentially 'empty' kilojoules
- they're better for your teeth.

An easy test of sugars versus starches is to eat a breakfast cereal made of puffed white rice and high in sugar. They're easy to find—just head for the kids' cereals! Time how long it is before you're hungry again. The next day, eat the same size serving of porridge or something else high in complex carbohydrates and fibre. I guarantee you will go much longer on the latter. A lunch test? Try a honey sandwich on white bread, versus a mixed-salad sandwich on multi-grain bread. No contest.

So, carbohydrates are 'good' and starches are the best. A large proportion of your daily fuel should come from complex, fibre-filled carbohydrates (about 55 per cent). This makes a balanced diet you can live with—happily and healthily—for the rest of your life.

GLYCAEMIC INDEX

The glycaemic index (GI) has received much attention and the term 'low GI' has crept into food labelling and marketing. GI is a rating system given to different sources of carbohydrates (sugars and starches) based on how quickly and how high they raise blood glucose after eating. This can be influenced by many factors, including how quickly they are digested and absorbed, whether they're simple or complex, how much fibre they contain, how processed or 'whole' the foods are, and preparation and cooking methods.

The glycaemic index of an individual food is measured against either pure glucose or white bread, both of which are given a GI value of 100. Foods which pass quickly into the bloodstream raise blood glucose quickly and are rated as high GI (>70). Medium-GI foods are ranked 56–69, and low-GI foods, which take longer to raise blood glucose, are below 55. Some foods you would assume to have a low GI (providing slow-release energy) are actually surprisingly high, such as white rice and potatoes, although sweet potatoes and pasta have lower values.

It is an interesting system, and is beneficial for people with diabetes, but there are problems associated with everyday application for the rest of us. A low GI rating does not necessarily mean a food is a healthier choice . . . Nutella rates much lower than watermelon, for example. GI gives no information of the *nutritional quality* or *energy density* of the food, which is what actually affects weight. Also, GI is measured on fasting patients eating individual foods, which is not how we eat in the real world. Once you eat meals in a non-fasting state, much of the GI differences are diminished.

GI gives us more information about how individual foods behave in the body, and has some important clinical applications. But in the real world, for most of us the exact numbers are not really important.

Protein

Protein yields about the same amount of energy as carbohydrates—about 17 kJ (4 Kcal) per gram. Proteins contain substances called amino acids, which are essential for building and repairing body tissues and making enzymes and hormones. There are 20 different amino acids, nine of which are called 'essential' as our body cannot make them, so we must obtain them from our food. Only animal products contain complete protein—in other words all the nine amino acids we need. Vegetarians need to choose a variety of grains and legumes to obtain them all.

The recommended daily intake of protein for women is 0.75 grams per kilo of body weight. This equates to 45 g for a 60 kg woman, for example. Pregnancy requires an extra 0.2 g/kg of protein (a total of 0.95 g/kg) during the last two trimesters, and 1.1 g/kg is recommended for breastfeeding.

Most Australians easily eat more than enough protein. Only rarely is extra protein required, even in cases of strenuous physical activity. Athletes generally need more total food, including good-quality protein, but expensive supplements are unnecessary. Our bodies do not need—and nor can they use—excessive amounts of protein. Surplus protein is broken down if not used as energy as it cannot be stored; the waste product (urea) is filtered out by the kidneys. Overloading on protein powders, bars and supplements just results in very expensive urine. Some other problems associated with high-protein diets include bone calcium loss and dehydration.

Protein usually only contributes 5–15 per cent of daily energy requirements, with carbohydrates and fats being the preferred energy sources. In extreme circumstances, such as anorexia or very low-energy diets, the body may be forced to break down muscle tissue (which is made of protein) for energy.

It is easy to get adequate quality protein from animal products such as eggs, dairy products, lean meat, chicken and fish. However, many animal sources of protein also contain a lot of saturated fat, so choose wisely. Chapter 5 has more about good options for protein.

Alcohol

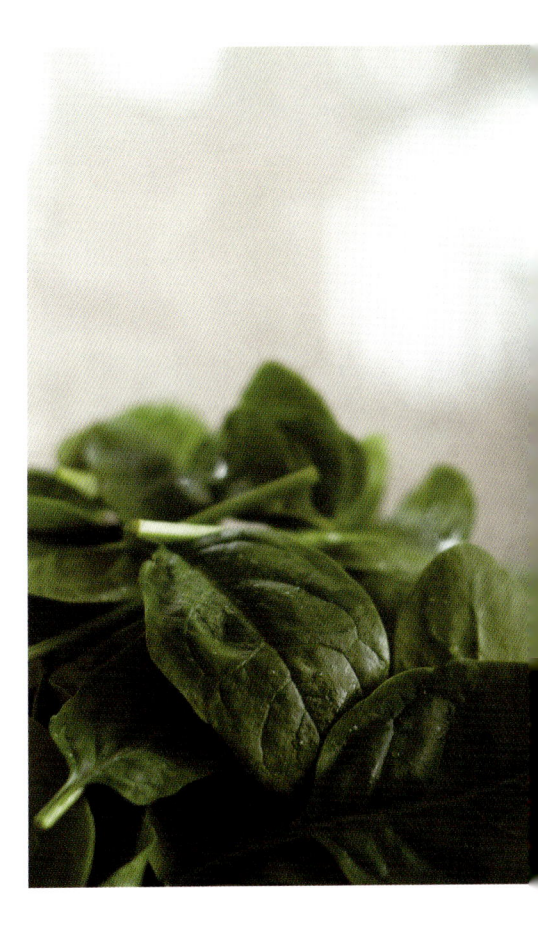

Alcohol provides about 29 kJ (7 Kcal) per gram—nearly as many kilojoules as fat. Alcohol also contains ethanol, which is toxic to nerve and muscle cells. At all times, your body will use the energy from alcohol first before protein, carbohydrate or fat because your body needs to get rid of it as quickly as possible. You do not store it and nor does it turn into fat.

A 'beer belly' is not made up of beer, but everything else that was eaten which wasn't used because the body was busy burning alcohol all the time. This means that if you drink a lot of alcohol, all the other energy you eat will be stored, and none of that extra body fat will budge while there are alcohol kilojoules to burn.

Another way alcohol works against you is in portion control. It is very easy to drink an exorbitant amount of kilojoules, particularly in social situations—but even if relaxing at home, after one drink, a second always follows easily . . . You're also likely to snack while drinking, and 'nibbles' like nuts, chips, dips and cheese plates are usually high in fat and may be followed by a meal too. Alcohol is the sneakiest fuel of all when it comes to excess empty kilojoules—lots of energy you have to burn, nothing good for the body, but it doesn't fill you up at all, so you still have to eat more food. If you drink alcohol regularly, you may find it difficult to use more energy than you consume.

The following tips will help ensure alcohol isn't sabotaging you.

- Save alcohol for special occasions while losing baby weight, and then consume only a moderate amount for weight maintenance.
- Don't drink every evening to relax. Pick one or two nights a week, like Friday or Sunday evening, sip and relish. Regularly using alcohol to escape or relax is a habit which will work against you. Drinking does not remove or help your stress, it simply masks it. Find other methods to relax—stretching, yoga, a walk, herbal tea, a shoulder or foot massage from your partner (ask for it!), a warm bath or listen to your favourite music through headphones if you need to tune out for a while. And don't forget you can also rev up to relax, because as you start to exercise, levels of endorphins ('feel-good' chemicals in the brain) rise and blood pressure lowers.
- At a party, drink mineral water first: it has bubbles, looks good in a flute, is great laced with fruit purée or juice and it quenches the thirst. By the time you get to the champagne you can just sip and savour. Also alternate water with alcoholic drinks to stop you drinking too much due to thirst. This helps counteract the dehydrating effects of alcohol as well.

- Watch out for creamy cocktails and sugary mixers such as soft drinks as they really rack up your kilojoule tally. Opt for soda or tonic mixers, fruit juice-based cocktails, or just have your drink 'on the rocks'. Or try a virgin cocktail or smoothie.
- If alcohol is one of the things you truly enjoy, buy the most expensive indulgence you can justify. Whatever your poison, from champagne to vodka, scotch or wine, you'll relish it and appreciate it—but you won't buy several rounds!
- Eat a decent meal before or with alcohol. You won't graze on fatty snacks and bottomless drinks all night at a function if you've had a good feed. It also slows down the absorption of alcohol, which means you won't get as intoxicated.

FUEL PREFERENCE AND WEIGHT CONTROL

We've established that alcohol, if present, is always the first choice of fuel used by your body as the body cannot store it. After that, the most readily available energy sources are glucose (broken-down carbohydrates) and fat in the bloodstream, and glycogen (stored carbohydrates) in muscles and the liver.

The last place your body looks for fuel is in the 'reserve tank' of stored body fat (adipose tissue). But as your physical activity gets more intense or longer in duration, your body uses fuel from muscles and stored fat in differing proportions. Chapter 7 looks more closely at fuel use in exercise.

A common pitfall in weight control is to 'advance purchase' a drinking or eating binge, rationalising that today's exercise session allows you excess kilojoules tonight. The problem is that the energy you used today came from what you ate and stored *yesterday* and *this morning*. The deal is, you have to burn off tonight's excesses tomorrow. So, have a wonderful meal out and enjoy all there is to offer. Why not, on occasion? But you'll need to add an extra kilometre or two on your walk the next day.

If you balance little splurges with extra physical activity, at the end of the week your energy balance can still work out even, or in deficit.

Remember: the body you have is a result of your lifestyle—and your lifestyle is a collection of habits . . . what you do *most of the time*. So if what you do most of the time is good for you, then you're well on the way to success.

Action

Find ways to move more

Use how your clothes fit as a guide to losing weight

Forget food fads

Limit alcohol consumption to when you'll really enjoy it, and don't binge. Pay for it the next day with exercise!

Look at the big picture—don't get bogged down in numbers and measuring everything . . . who's got the time, anyway?

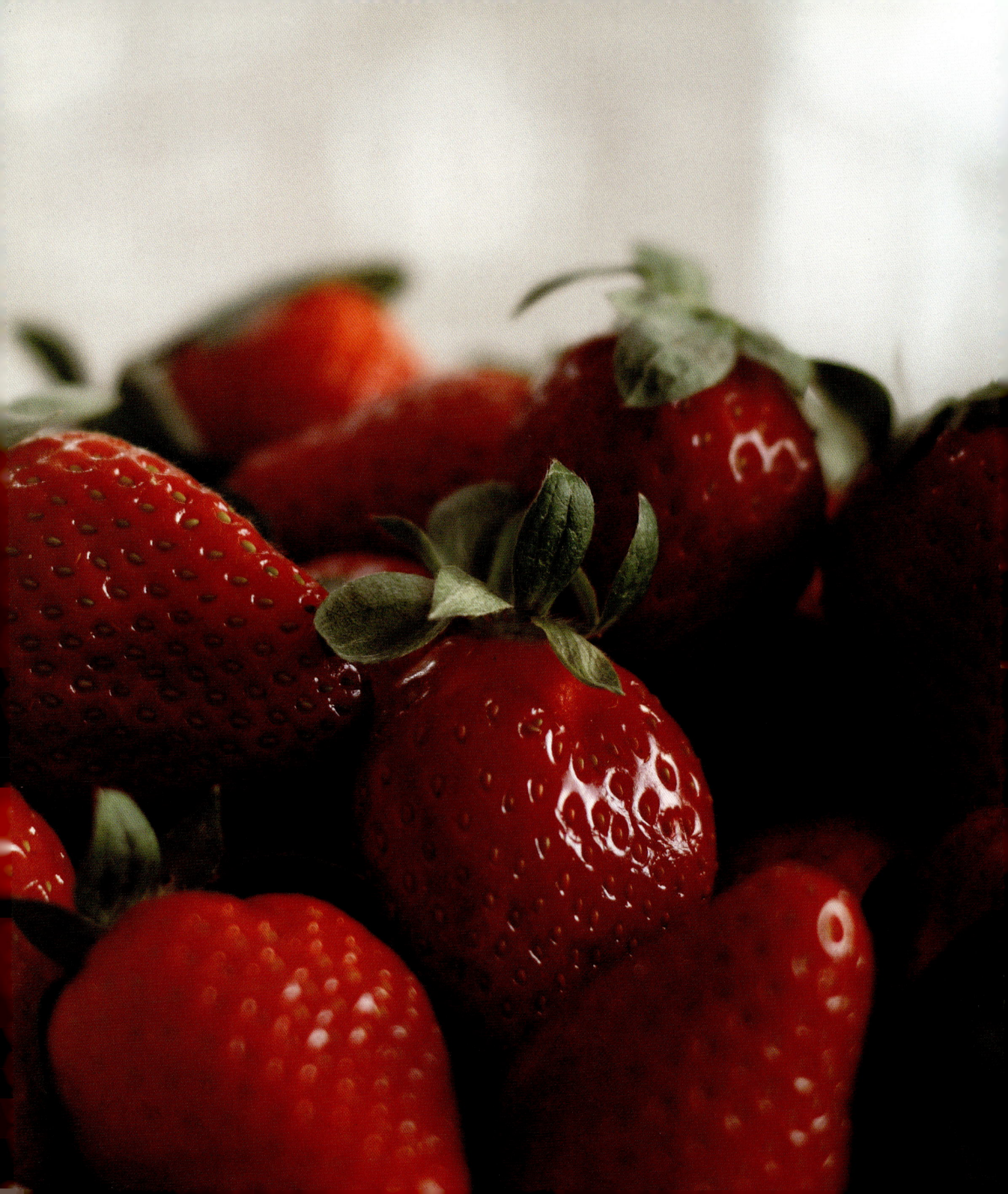

Food for body and soul

Most people know what constitutes good nutrition and they know what they *should* eat. They also say it's too hard to be healthy, that they don't have time to cook or plan meals. So every time a quick-fix comes along, they subscribe in the hope it is a shortcut to good health and weight loss. But I suspect that, as a mother, you're ready to cut the nonsense. You're ready to admit that the little voice in your head, who tells you to get off the couch and eat well, is actually trying to help you.

Food is pleasure. We all have the right to enjoy eating without guilt. How often do you feel guilty about something you eat? Every week, every day, every meal? Why is it all your food vices, indulgences or pleasures are 'bad' for you? Why do you want to *over*indulge in chocolate or chips? Women often refer to being 'weak' when it comes to certain foods, claiming 'I really shouldn't' when offered some cake. When you're in control you can have some cake and eat it too. You don't go overboard and you don't feel guilty. You are accountable for it. You balance it into your weekly energy intake and expenditure. Of course, there will be fewer indulgences if they are particularly energy rich and you're trying to lose weight. But positive, optimal eating and taking control of your habits and your nutrition eliminates guilt, while allowing gastronomic pleasures—for life.

Does it sound too good to be true? It isn't.

How much time do you spend preoccupied with food, diets or weight? Even if it's only three minutes of every waking hour (let's pretend you sleep eight hours, ha!) this could add up to 48 minutes over a 16-hour day. If you spent 48 minutes each day collecting healthy food ideas from magazines, planning meals, exercising, or learning about nutrition or physiology, you'd never have to wonder whether a diet will work again! A daily exercise session of 48 minutes could tip the energy equation in your favour and solve your weight issues for good.

Ready?

Forget dieting for good and start eating positively

Life is too short to live without chocolate—but too long to eat the whole box!

Get savvy about good nutrition

Identify foods and drinks that sabotage weight loss

Quality over quantity nurtures body and soul—every time

Still not working? Check your food portions!

DO NOT DIET BECAUSE . . .

Even if a diet does work in the short term, the results are rarely evident a year later, and a significant proportion of dieters will put on more weight than before the diet. The human body is very resilient and adaptable and our bodies often overreact for self-preservation. As described in chapter 4, when energy intake is restricted, the body responds by slowing energy use to preserve it for vital functions. That is, our metabolic rate slows and we store more. Then when you give up the restricted eating, your body piles on the weight, even if you're eating less than before the diet. In a way, it's nice to know your body is trying to save you, not ruin your efforts. But it's more important to remember how it works so you can plan weight-loss tactics accordingly.

Meal-replacement shakes, drinks, powders and bars are a marketing trap. They are expensive, unsustainable, unnecessary and terrible for your metabolism. If you do lose weight on these meal replacements, chances are you will suffer side effects ranging from nausea to kidney stress, constipation and fatigue.

Instead, right now, you can eat well, treat your body well and live without dieting. Commit to it for yourself and your family and then do what it takes—learn about nutrition from reliable sources, prioritise your health and apply the knowledge. It need not be a lifelong struggle—it's simply a choice, every day.

With young children, you do not have the time, inclination, focus or energy to stick to a strict diet. The constant demands for baby's feeds and toddler's meals are taxing enough without having to cook a separate 'diet' meal for yourself and then something 'real' for your partner, who is probably working overtime too! You may be sleep deprived and cannot risk nutritional deficiencies as well. You must eat well for health, energy, immunity and strength for the marathon of pregnancy, childbirth, breastfeeding and the years beyond. As all mums know, there's just no down time on this job.

Diets mess with your head, your moods, your stability, your confidence and self-esteem. Diets create a nasty cocktail of stress, deprivation, excessive effort, bingeing, guilt, denial, frustration, failure—not a great model for a healthy lifestyle. And that's exactly what you are to your children: they learn by example, not from what you say, but what you *do*. A mother who is obsessed with food and weight issues, and is negative about her body, sends an unhealthy message to her children. A friend was shocked to see her preschooler mimic her on the bathroom scales, saying her four-year-old frame was fat and disgusting. Remember, you set the tone for nutrition and exercise for your children. Healthy eating, exercise habits and food preparation skills give children the one gift without which they can do little: lifelong health.

POSITIVE EATING FOR GOOD NUTRITION

You can lose the baby weight by taking positive, optimal steps rather than by sacrificing yourself to negative restriction and denial—by focusing on what to eat and what to do, instead of what not to do. Positive eating is all about finding the best nourishment for *you*, both physically and emotionally.

The first step in positive eating is to understand what your body really needs and can use. Chapter 4 detailed the three nutrients we use for fuel, repair and building: carbohydrates, proteins and fats. The other three essential nutrients are water, vitamins and minerals.

I remember learning about the Good Food Pyramid at school. It's not sexy, it's not flashy, it makes no comments about weight loss, yet nutritionists keep coming back to it because it's accurate, it works and it's sustainable. Now, to avoid labelling foods as 'good' or 'bad', Nutrition Australia uses the Healthy Eating Pyramid (you can view it online at www.nutritionaustralia.org). There are many different forms of this model, but they all essentially say the same thing. The pyramid model does not address kilojoule intake, serving sizes or food portions; it represents *proportion*. So, in contrast to recent fad diets which may be low in carbohydrate, high in protein or moderate in fat, the Healthy Eating Pyramid expresses what nutritionists have been saying for decades:

Eat most: vegetables, dried peas, beans, lentils, cereals, bread, fruit, nuts—this group contains mostly complex carbohydrates, as well as some protein and fat sources.

Eat moderately: lean meat, eggs, fish, skinless chicken, milk, yoghurt, cheese—this group is high in protein, but also contains some carbohydrate and fat.

Eat in small amounts: oil, margarine, reduced-fat spreads, butter, sugar—this group contains mostly fat, plus some simple sugar (carbohydrate).

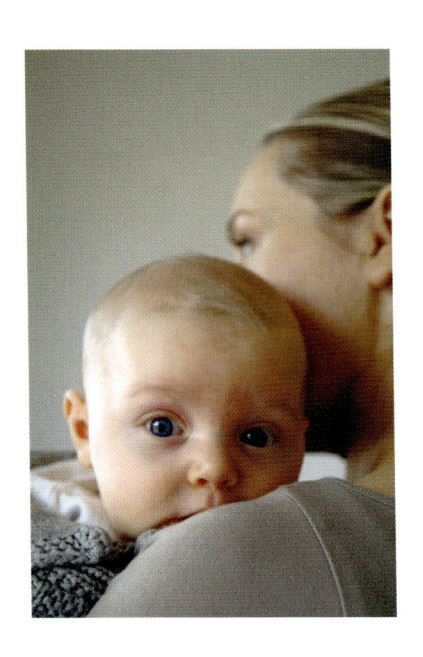

In this triangular model, the 'eat most' section forms the base of the pyramid, 'eat moderately' is in the middle and 'eat in small amounts' forms the very tip. This is enough information for me. No-one divides, weighs, measures and then compares each nutrient in each meal to determine daily percentage intakes, every day. Would you even *want* to do that? How would you analyse a casserole without a laboratory at home? Sometimes more detail is just more. I'm all about practicality and keeping it simple.

Using the pyramid recommendations you can easily determine to which group the foods you usually eat belong. For example, your cereals or grains include rice, corn, wheat, oats and barley, but also pasta, couscous, semolina, amaranth, kamut, millet, quinoa, rye, spelt, teff and buckwheat. Look, I've never tried some of these either, but there are a lot of interesting, healthy and delicious choices if you start to look. Of course, all dairy products belong in the 'eat moderately' category except butter, cream and ice cream, which are 'eat in small amounts'.

The proportions can be related to the day or to a single meal. So, if you have a meal made only of ice cream and cake (kids' parties!) then for the rest of your day you should focus on the other food groups. If you're building a sandwich, have mostly bread and salad with some lean protein like a slice of turkey or cheese and top it off with a dab of dressing or mayonnaise . . . and it's your perfect pyramid lunch. Apply the same proportions to your dinner plate. Too easy.

The beauty of the pyramid's simplicity is that the proportions are applicable throughout your life—for children, during pregnancies and breastfeeding, and later in life.

Below is my own 'Lifestyle Pyramid', with example meals and foods (rather than ingredients). Since we are made up of what we eat *most* of the time, make sure your intake is heavy with the first category.

Eat most: anything that is grown in the ground or picked from a plant (in its most natural, least processed form), and fresh, simple home-prepared meals.

Eat moderately: animal products, healthier takeaway or commercially prepared foods (these do exist and all busy mums need options).

Eat in small amounts: unhealthy, fatty fast foods/takeaway, junk food or 'treats' such as sweets, chips, biscuits, cakes, ice cream, highly manufactured meat products such as hot dogs and some deli meats, anything deep-fried.

The National Heart Foundation recommends fat intake should be less than 30 per cent of total daily kilojoules, of which saturated (animal) fats make up less than 10 per cent. Nutritionists generally recommend that a further 15–20 per cent of our energy should come from protein, and the remaining 50–55 per cent from carbohydrate.

Another way to look at it is the recommended servings:

- 4–9 serves of bread, grains, cereal, rice, pasta, etc.
- 4–5 serves of vegetables
- 2–3 serves of fruit
- 2 serves of milk, yoghurt, cheese
- 1–2 serves of meat, poultry, fish, legumes, eggs or nuts.

Remember, suggested servings are always for the 'average' person, and how often does one size really fit all? It is the relative proportions which are more important and easy enough to perceive.

The exact number of total kilojoules you need to consume varies widely depending on your height, weight, body composition, fitness level, age and activity level during the day. Table 5.1 shows guidelines from the federal government's Healthy Active website to give you an idea of the ranges.

If you are 31, for example, average in size and do no physical activity or are bed-ridden, you may require around 7300 kJ a day, whereas an elite athlete may need closer to 12,500 kJ. If you're an average mum, running around toddlers with some part-time work squeezed in and a half-hour walk with the pram to the shops for dinner supplies, then you'll require something in between the two extremes.

Vitamins, minerals and fibre

The food pyramid is designed so you don't need to remember what every vitamin and mineral is for and how to get it; if intake is balanced as suggested, and your diet is varied, it is hard to be deficient in anything. The same goes for fibre: from the 'eat most' group you'll get plenty of insoluble fibre which sweeps out the insides, and soluble fibre which helps lower cholesterol. And the 'eat moderately' group will also cover calcium and iron. The food diary exercise in chapter 6 is useful to check if your diet is well balanced and varied enough. If you have real concerns from there about specific nutrient intakes, consult a nutritionist, dietician or your doctor.

TABLE 5.1
Estimated kJ/day for females to maintain a healthy weight (ranging from sedentary to active lifestyles)

AGE (YEARS)	KJ PER DAY
19–30	7100–13,900
31–50	7300–12,500
51–70	6900–12,000
70+	5600–11,500

(www.healthyactive.gov.au)

Remember that vitamin and mineral supplements have not been proven to help anything other than diseases specifically caused by deficiencies. There are certain groups of the population at risk of deficiency who may benefit from supplementation, such as those with digestive disorders or the elderly, but for everyone else it is hard to be deficient. And also keep in mind that too much of anything can become toxic in the body. For example, excessive vitamin A is particularly dangerous during pregnancy as it can cause birth defects.

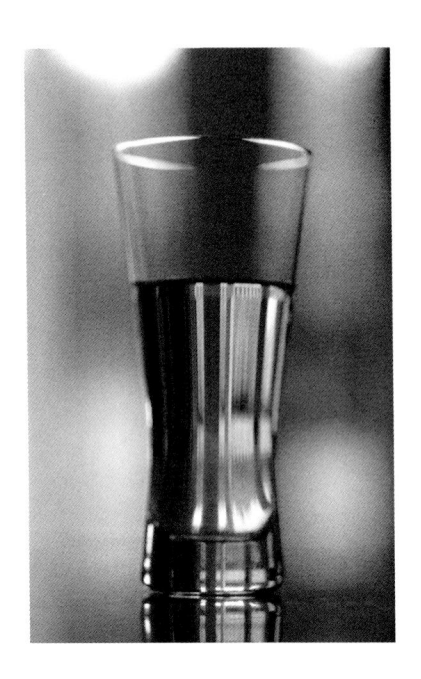

Water

Water is a vital nutrient involved in practically every physiological reaction and process in the body. It plays an essential role in general health, fitness and body composition goals.

The exact amount of water we need varies according to factors like body size and composition, activity level and diet. An easy guide to whether you're drinking enough water is urine colour: anything darker than pale straw and you need more. As a guide, eight glasses (two litres) a day is generally recommended, which can include water contained in food and other drinks. Pregnant and breastfeeding mothers need more due to increased blood volume (which can increase by 50 per cent during pregnancy) and milk requirements. Exercise and warm weather also increase requirements.

Drinking water is one of the best things you can do for your health, for many reasons beyond hydration. Other drinks provide water, but also additives your body may not need, such as extra kilojoules, sugar, chemicals, preservatives, flavours and colours. Most people do not drink enough water, which can have the following effects.

- Symptoms ranging from headaches and nausea in the short term, to dry skin and kidney problems in the long term.
- Without sufficient water, carbohydrate energy will not be stored in the muscles for exercise—carbohydrates cannot be stored without water, but fat can, which can work against your weight-loss plans.
- The vital process of regulating body temperature can be seriously impaired (just like in your car, water is used to dissipate heat—blood vessels carry the blood closer to the surface of the skin for cooling).

Here are some tips for getting and staying properly hydrated.

- Basically drink as much water as possible—many people eat or overeat when they are actually thirsty.
- Keep a glass of water beside the kitchen sink and have a small drink whenever you pass through.
- Whenever you're out, carry a water bottle with you—you've probably got a bag full of snacks, wipes, drinks and nappies anyway, so what's one more bottle?
- Drink a glass of water before each meal, and sip water throughout. Also, drink half a glass of water before you reach for any snack—you will feel fuller and tend not to eat as much.
- Have a glass of water as soon as you wake up in the morning because sleep is very dehydrating, especially if you're in a temperature-controlled environment.
- Limit caffeine intake in coffee, tea or soft drinks. It is a diuretic, which causes water loss through urine.
- Don't drink fruit juice to quench thirst—and especially never 'fruit drinks', which contain added sugars, flavours, colours, preservatives and lots of empty kilojoules. Pure fruit juice is high in natural fruit sugars (fructose), so you can drink a lot of kilojoules in a couple of glasses of juice a day. Water quenches thirst without kilojoules. Children also should not get used to juice as a regular drink—it is bad for their teeth and trains them to want sweet drinks. It is much healthier to eat the fruit the juice came from and get the fibre, vitamins and satiety as well, rather than lots of quick kilojoules.
- Avoid soft drinks. They have loads of kilojoules in the form of refined sugar, as well as lots of nasty chemicals, artificial flavours, preservatives and even caffeine. Don't drink 'diet' soft drinks either because they contain even more chemicals, and only feed our taste for the overly sweet. Also, 'diet' soft drinks don't work. Several recent studies have shown people who drink diet soft drinks are more overweight and less successful on diets than those who drink regular soft drinks because they overcompensate with food—they figure they can have the mudcake with cream because they've chosen the 'diet' drink!

If you really have to have something different or special to drink instead of plain water, try sparkling mineral water on its own, or with a dash of fruit juice, fruit purée or passionfruit pulp. Or try iced water with a slice of lemon or lime, or drink out of a chilled wine or champagne glass. These can help enhance the experience and the taste.

Also weigh yourself directly before and after exercising to determine how much water you've lost. Weight loss indicates water lost through perspiration as well as from carbohydrate stores used for energy. Digital scales are best for this. If there is a difference of 300 grams, for example, that means a net water loss of 300 millilitres, which you need to replace. Don't forget to sip water throughout your workout to prevent dehydration as well—even while swimming.

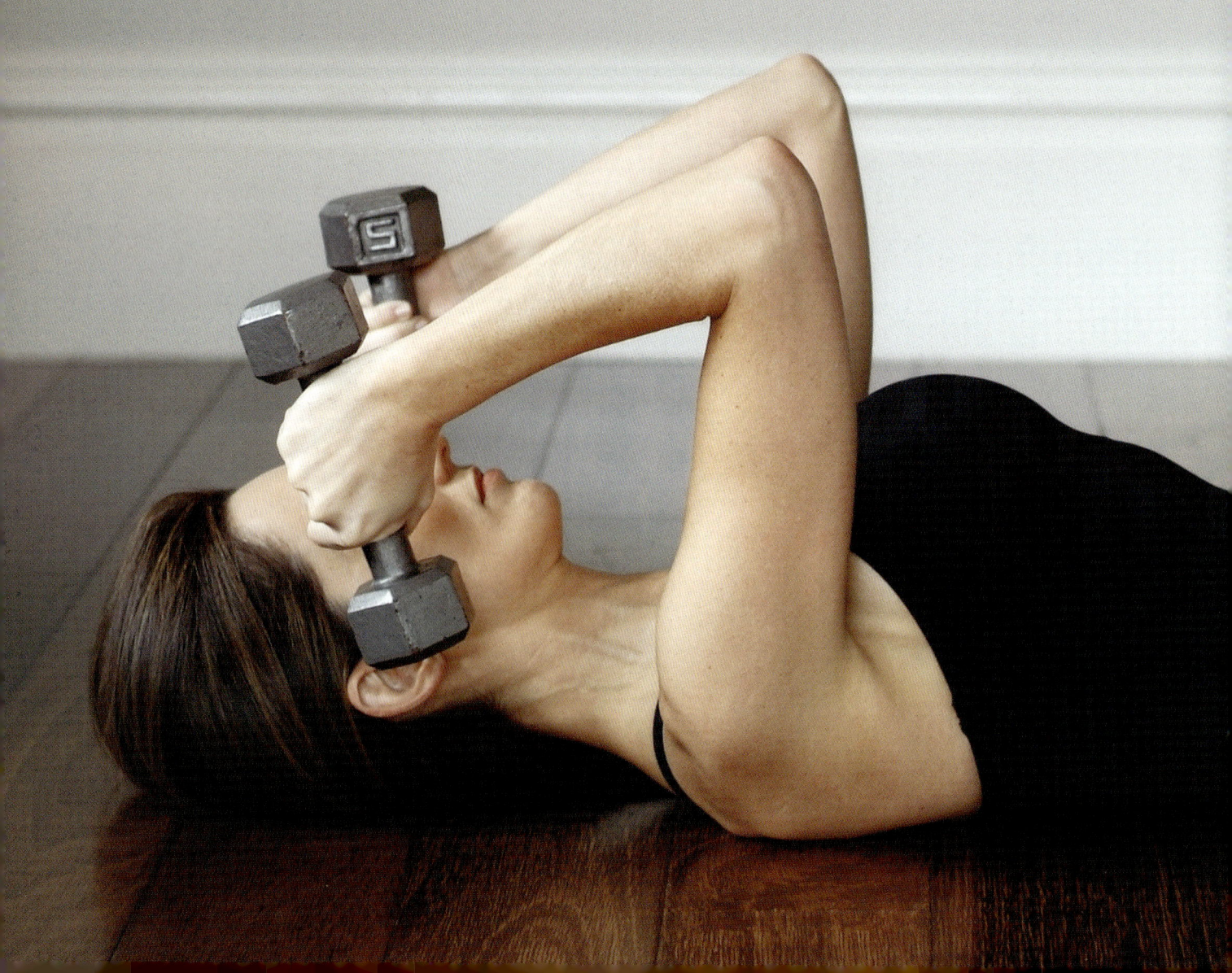

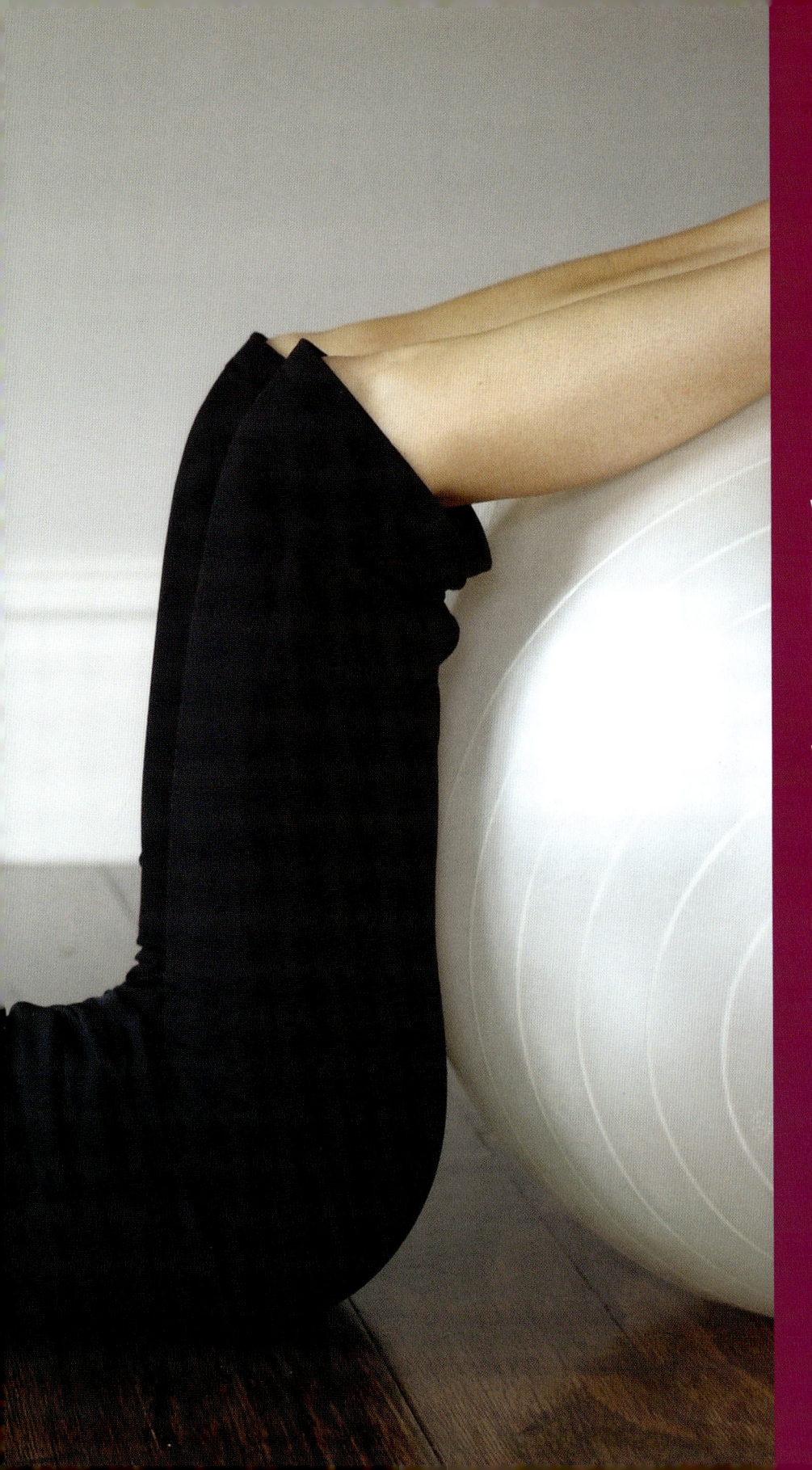

'You did what you knew how to do, and when you knew better, you did better'

Maya Angelou

FOOD FOR BODY AND SOUL 73

Some people complain that drinking lots of water sends them to the toilet too often. The only way to adapt is to keep doing it and your body will respond. As you get fitter, your lean tissues and capillary networks increase to store water and supply blood, making many body functions more efficient. Fitter muscles store carbohydrate energy more efficiently (and more water along with it), and all your organs, including your skin, will have a much richer supply of water and oxygen.

Breastfeeding mums

The food pyramid model still applies to women who are breastfeeding. Breastfeeding mums require an extra 2000–2100 kJ (480–500 Kcal) per day for milk production (for full breastfeeding during the first six months, and then partial). This is a rough guide, as there are so many variables: some women produce a little milk and supplement it with formula, some women have litres of milk to spare. Some women feed for only a few weeks, some for a couple of years. Some women start feeding with lots of stored energy (body fat), some have little. But as a general rule, the energy requirements are a little more than during pregnancy if you're feeding fulltime.

Listen to your body and if you're really hungry eat a bit more, but don't go overboard, particularly if you want to start losing some baby weight. As mentioned in chapter 4, the recommended protein intake for breastfeeding is 1.1 g/kg body weight. As for the other nutrients, if you're eating a little more of everything and your diet is varied and balanced with lots of fresh fruit and vegies, you'll be fine.

You can safely lose weight while breastfeeding, so long as it's not drastic or fast—around two kilos per month is generally fine. A steady loss with good nutrition and exercise shouldn't affect milk production. Drastic diets can compromise your milk supply, and remember that you're already using extra energy and your metabolic rate is up to make the milk, so this already tips the energy equation in your favour. If you can't seem to lose all the weight you want in the first nine to 12 months after the birth, don't worry about the last few kilos until after you stop feeding. After a year the weight should get easier to lose even if you're still feeding, as baby gets an increasing proportion of nutrients from food, and breast milk is relegated to 'supplement' status.

The Australian government's *Australian Guide to Healthy Eating*

(www.healthyactive.gov.au) recommends the following servings per day during breastfeeding:
- 5–7 serves of bread, grains, cereals, rice, pasta
- 7 serves of vegetables, legumes
- 5 serves of fruit
- 2 serves of milk, yoghurt, cheese
- 2 serves of meat, fish, poultry, eggs, nuts and legumes.

Breastfeeding also requires a higher water intake. Sip while feeding and drink with meals; you need about nine glasses a day!

YOUR BODY IS A TEMPLE—TREAT IT WELL

The success of healthy eating depends entirely on fitting it into your lifestyle. You don't want or need someone telling you exactly what to eat for the rest of your life. Use the following guidelines as a checklist for food management. Implement the small steps and strategies and let them become habit. They are relatively simple, but effective.

Golden rules for eating

- Breakfast like a queen, lunch like a princess, dine like a pauper. Never skip the queen's meal, breakfast. You need energy for the day and you are more likely to use the energy from this meal than store it.
- Eat five times a day. That's right: breakfast, lunch and dinner, with two snacks in between. This keeps energy levels constant for busy and breastfeeding mums. It also keeps your metabolism revving along so your body doesn't panic and store energy. Having more frequent, smaller meals keeps your blood sugar more stable and prevents excessive hunger, making you less likely to overeat and make poor food choices. You don't need a meal for snacks. In fact you don't need a meal every meal; it can just be food—not 'cuisine'. Chances are you already snack between meals—most people do. They don't intend to eat until dinner, but are starving by 5 p.m. and start on the chips and dips. So pay attention to what you're really eating and make a positive choice.
- Don't eat after dinner. I have this rule for my toddlers. Once they leave the table, that's it. No snacks at bedtime. If my toddlers can

do it, so can you. You don't need energy at night; unless you're going dancing, you'll store it. Enjoy a relaxing herbal tea before bed if you need something.

- ❖ Dessert is also something you don't need. Save this one for special dinners out. You can eat the kilojoule content of your dinner again on a dessert plate, every night! Dessert is just a habit. Appetisers are another habit which can further multiply your dinner. Just eat dinner; you don't need three courses every night. If you want something sweet, have some fruit with dinner, but don't treat it as another meal, waiting for dinner to 'go down' to fit it in.

Soul food

Which foods would you choose for your last meal on a deserted island? I love mangoes, I love seafood and I *love* chocolate. Two out of three are good for my body; the other is great for my soul. Keep your 'soul food' on the list. If I went a week without chocolate I'd be capable of eating a whole block before I made it to the supermarket checkout!

Don't pick all your favourites, just the ones you'd really miss. Most of us have a few favourites we know aren't contributing to good health and may be causing excess weight. So eat these less desirable foods, *in small amounts*, when you want. Moderation is the key. It's much wiser and easier to get in shape a little more slowly and enjoy it, rather than deny yourself everything you love, then fail.

The French really know how to feed the soul. Even the simplest lunch of a freshly baked baguette—crisp on the outside, light and soft in the middle—with sharp, creamy, perfectly aged cheese and sweet, rich red, sun-ripened tomatoes is an unparalleled delight, executed with effortless attention to simple quality. Compare this to the average cheese and tomato sandwich from your local takeaway: a highly processed, pre-wrapped square of bland, manufactured cheese and pale, flavourless tomato on a perfectly square piece of preservative-laden white bread.

Quality over quantity will feed the soul every time. If you really enjoy a meal—if it has real taste, flavour, texture, colour and aroma—you will not feel deprived. We have a great range of fresh produce of excellent quality in our country; when bought in season, it is more affordable than processed and packaged foods—another good reason to indulge in quality.

Your soul food needs to be savoured to be fully appreciated and to

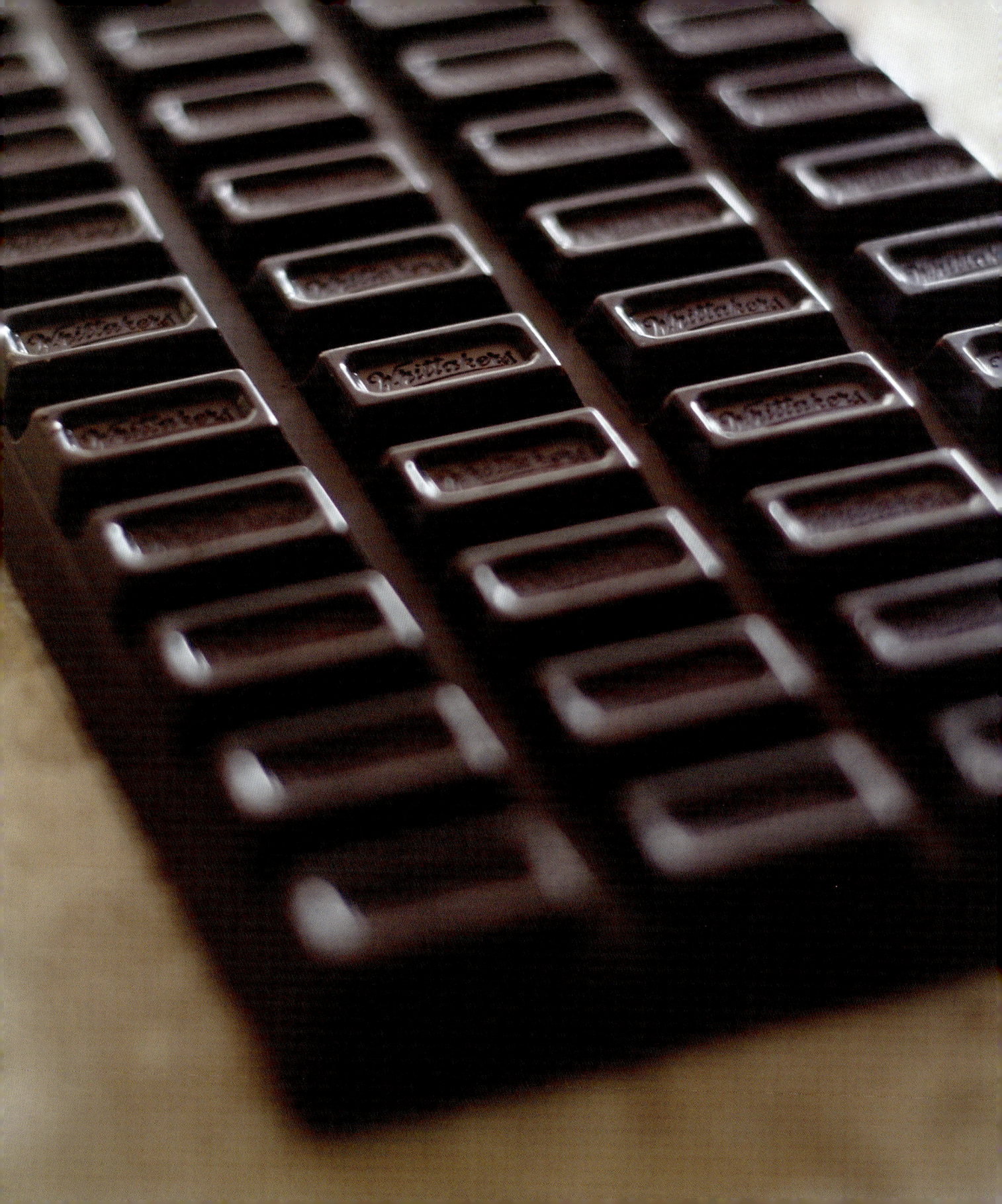

satisfy. It is no good standing at the fridge scoffing down biscuits! Having something 'special' helps keep you on track 'most of the time', which is what really counts. Here's how to enjoy feeding the soul.

- Pay attention to the little things that can make everyday meals an experience. Eat meals seated at the table with proper utensils.
- For family meals together, light candles or put flowers on the table. Everyone will feel special, even if it's just spaghetti bolognaise again.
- Don't eat meals in front of the television or standing at the refrigerator. It's too easy to overeat or forget these meals.
- If you have a special treat, slow down and be in the moment. Savour the flavour, and enjoy the texture in every bite. Don't have your indulgence while multi-tasking; you may not even notice it! Your treat can be a ritual, so long as it is reasonably sized, not too frequent, satisfies you and really feeds your soul.

TABLE 5.2

JUNK FOODS	BETTER CHOICES
Chips	Pretzels, rice crackers, air-popped popcorn
Prepared creamy dips	Salsa, home-made light sour cream dips
Sweets, lollies	Dried fruits, nuts, cereals
Ice cream	Fresh or frozen low-fat yoghurt
Sweet biscuits, cakes, doughnuts, muffins	Fruit, rice cakes or toast with 100 per cent fruit jam, home-made low-fat mini muffins, 'healthy' biscuits (check the label)
Chocolate	There's no suitable substitute! But tread lightly . . .
Frozen commercial pizza	A quick, simple home-made pizza

Junk food

I don't like labelling food as bad or good. Instead, think in terms of 'everyday' food and 'sometimes' food. Remember, it's not about banning foods, it's about positive choices and eating optimally *most* of the time.

Junk food is 'sometimes' food that is excessively high in kilojoules, may hold little nutritional value, is often addictive and doesn't satisfy hunger. Try these more optimal substitutes (or think of your own) for foods you really don't want in your regular diet (see Table 5.2 for a few ideas). You may be surprised how little you miss them!

CHECK FOOD LABELS

Healthy fresh food does wonders for your body. Try to eat as few packaged, processed or manufactured foods as possible—that way there is no question what you're really getting: an apple contains 100 per cent apple, a salmon steak is 100 per cent salmon. When you shop for food, fill your basket mostly with items from the produce section (just like the food pyramid). If your basket contains mostly boxes and packets, you need to rethink what you're buying.

It is also vital to understand food labels. Nutrition Australia has comprehensive information about food labels on their website (www.nutritionaustralia.org). The important points to look for on food labels are:

- **Ingredients:** you'd be surprised what's actually in processed foods if you've never read the labels. Ingredients are always listed in descending order of quantity, so the first ingredient is present in the largest amount. If the first ingredient is not what you are intending to buy, reconsider. For example, if you're buying a fruit preserve and the first ingredient is sugar, and fruit is somewhere way down the list, shop around.
- **Artificial additives:** choose products with the fewest added colours, flavours and preservatives, particularly if you're breastfeeding. This can be as simple as choosing cheese which needs refrigeration, instead of one which can live in the pantry.
- **Energy:** the kilojoules 'per serving' may be of interest later at home, but when you're charging around the grocery store, a teary toddler in the trolley and a baby strapped to your chest, the quickest way to assess a food is to look at the 'per 100 g' column. This clearly shows the relative proportions of the nutrients in the food. So, if this column says six grams of fat, the food contains 6 per cent fat. Some foods naturally contain a high percentage of fat, like oils, butter and nuts, but it's the sneaky fats or extra sugar added to enhance a food's palatability or texture that you need to look out for.

Always keep in mind that whatever you eat today, you carry around as part of you tomorrow—whether it's fat, sugar, chemicals or preservatives. So choose foods based on your goals of optimal health for the whole family.

PORTION CONTROL

Let's assume you're now eating a healthy, fresh, balanced diet most of the time. It is possible you are still not losing weight. Remember our basic energy equation: if you eat more energy than you use, you will gain weight. Recall that fat has more kilojoules than other nutrients—so if you reduce your fat intake, but not necessarily your food portions, you reduce total kilojoules (energy).

Still not losing weight? Move more.

Can't move enough to move the weight? Managing food portions is the next nutritional step to losing weight without 'dieting'.

If you have become disconnected from the messages your body gives you when you're full, you'll have trouble keeping hunger at bay and will have to relearn the way you eat. I won't recommend you weigh and measure food, because even I wouldn't do that.

Our learned behaviours become our eating habits, our automatic choices. We can change these by *consciously* being aware of these habits and choosing better options. If you are used to eating a full plate, then having another serving, you can replace this habit with ones that control your portions. Here's how.

- Drink more water—this is the number-one, kilojoule-free way to curb appetite. Drink between meals, and particularly before and during meals. You'll feel fuller and stay hydrated.
- Eat more slowly. Let the food digest, let nutrients absorb into the bloodstream, let the stomach feel full and your body will tell you when you've had enough. If it's all inhaled in less than five minutes none of this will have time to register. Eat like my children: their meals last a good hour as they can hardly get the food in between all the chatter!
- Choose fibrous starches and lean, quality protein, which make you feel fuller and take longer to process than simple sugars.
- Don't save all your protein for dinner. Have a good serving at breakfast or lunch to get you through the day. When feeling tired on the afternoon stretch, we scavenge for high-energy snacks. A good dose of protein at lunch and a healthy, planned snack will prevent the afternoon blow-out.
- Don't snack or sample as you cook. If you've eaten regularly throughout the day and had a decent afternoon snack and drink,

you shouldn't be starving as you cook. Seal foods as they're ready; sabotage the ingredients if you must. For example, if you're preparing a chicken and vegie stir-fry, pile the raw chicken on top of the rest of the food (providing it will be cooked later, of course). You couldn't possibly pick at this! This is a way of controlling an unwanted behaviour by replacing it with an incompatible behaviour. Or try chewing a stick of sugar-free gum or even brushing your teeth before cooking.

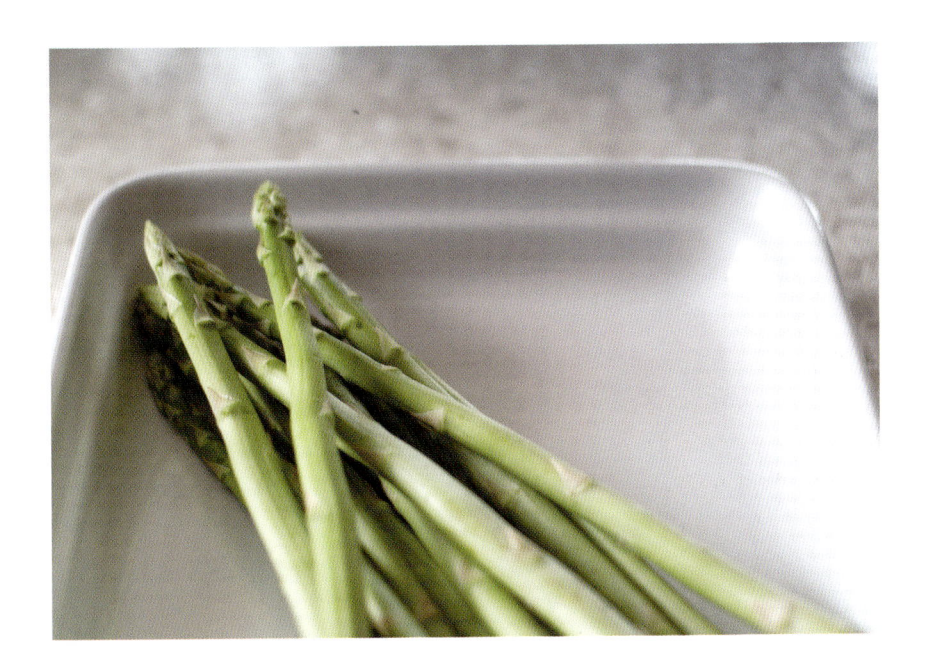

❖ This one baffles me and it's really common: many mothers have told me they finish their children's meals because they hate to waste so much food. The situation is: you've served it, they've picked over it, they didn't finish it, and it's between you or the bin. Do you really want your body to be a substitute for the bin? The pre-chewed, finger-puppeted, sneezed-on contents of my children's dinner plates could not hold less appeal for me! But some women polish off anything their child doesn't eat, either as an excuse to snack or most likely as a subconscious act. Paying attention to what happens to the food during the meal is a starting point to avoiding eating it. Children stop eating when they're full and shouldn't be made to finish everything. Who decides what a serving or a plateful is? The appropriate serving is one which satisfies hunger, not what is dished out by the kitchen, at home or elsewhere. So, allowing your children to stop when they are full is important for them to develop a healthy relationship with food. If they are constantly wasting a lot, stop serving so much! Serve a little: if they devour it, give them more. Any left over that wasn't served? Refrigerate it: this will save you time tomorrow. Give them variety; try new things. Be creative with picky eaters, and try things over and over, in different ways. Trying foods regularly, in small amounts, will help sneak it into their diets eventually.

- Reduce portions by using smaller dishes—you'll feel less deprived with a smaller heaped plate than a relatively empty large plate. Your body size could be predetermined by the size of your dinner set! Large plates make large people: have you visited an American-style steakhouse recently? Using a smaller plate or bowl automatically reduces serving size and allows you to stop, think, have a drink and check if you really are hungry before a second helping.
- Never eat directly out of the fridge or cupboard, or from a box, bag or carton, or in front of the television.
- Eating out is a treat—not an excuse to overindulge. Instead of three courses, try ordering two entrees and a hot drink to finish. That way you won't sit with an empty placemat while others have every course. If it's a buffet, use the smaller bread plate and choose wisely. Fill up on fresh fruit and vegetables, lean protein and starches which slow you down after the first plate. Starting off small and going slowly will let you digest, have a drink and register fullness before going back for more. At social functions, the key is to focus on being social, not on eating. Plan ahead and eat something satisfying beforehand, so you won't ravenously inhale every passing hors d'oeuvre tray.

This chapter has provided the basic framework for your new lifestyle, outlining nutritional guidelines and positive goals for optimal health. The next chapter helps you apply these to your own individual lifestyle with minimal disruption or sacrifice.

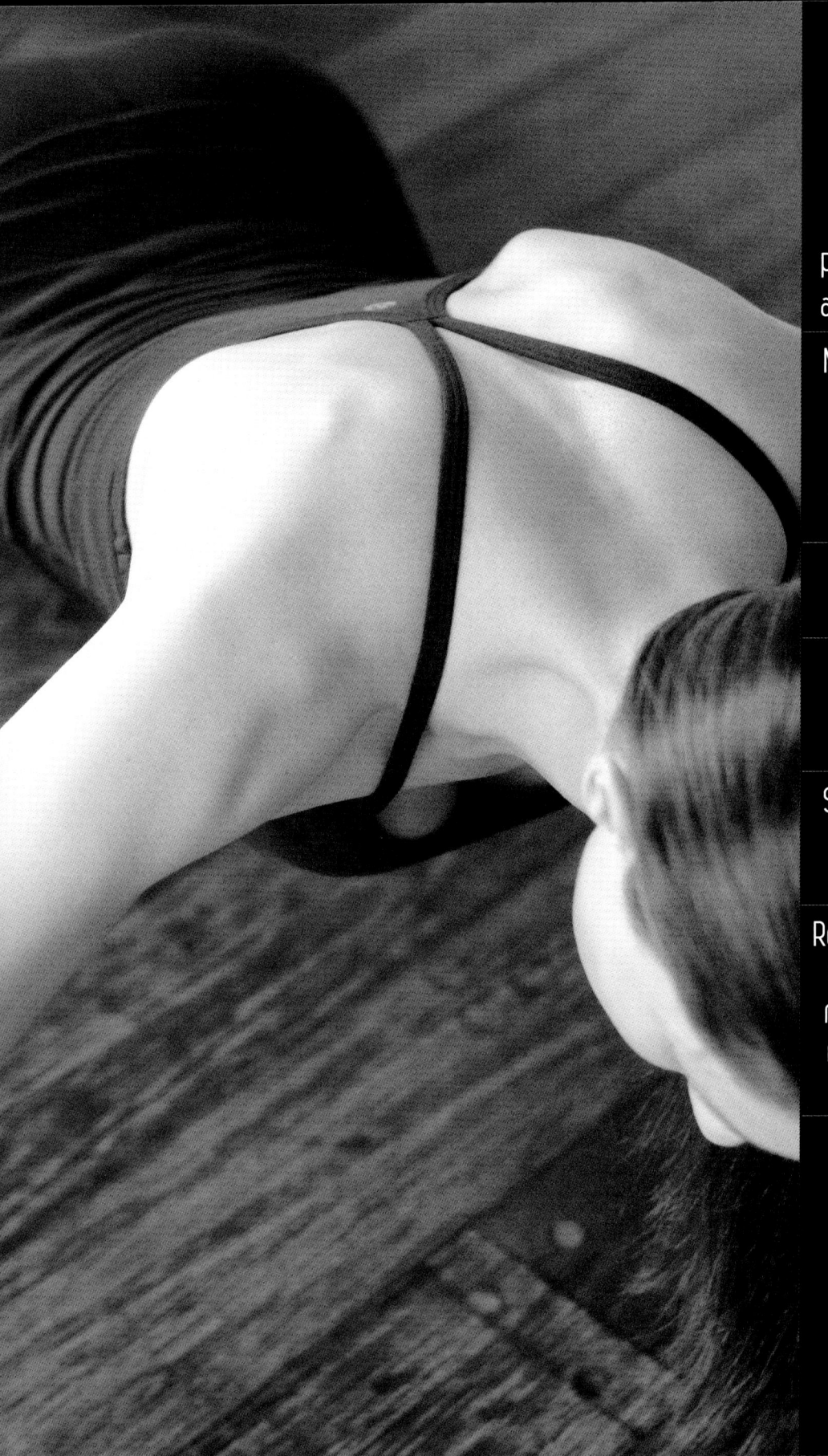

Action

Pack up your diet books and magazines for good

Make a list of the foods you like which fit into the food pyramid categories and keep expanding this list

Find ways to drink lots of water

Take the time to stop and enjoy your meals and your life

Start making conscious food choices based on positive eating

Read food labels—finding the best products will make your shopping so much quicker, simpler and better informed

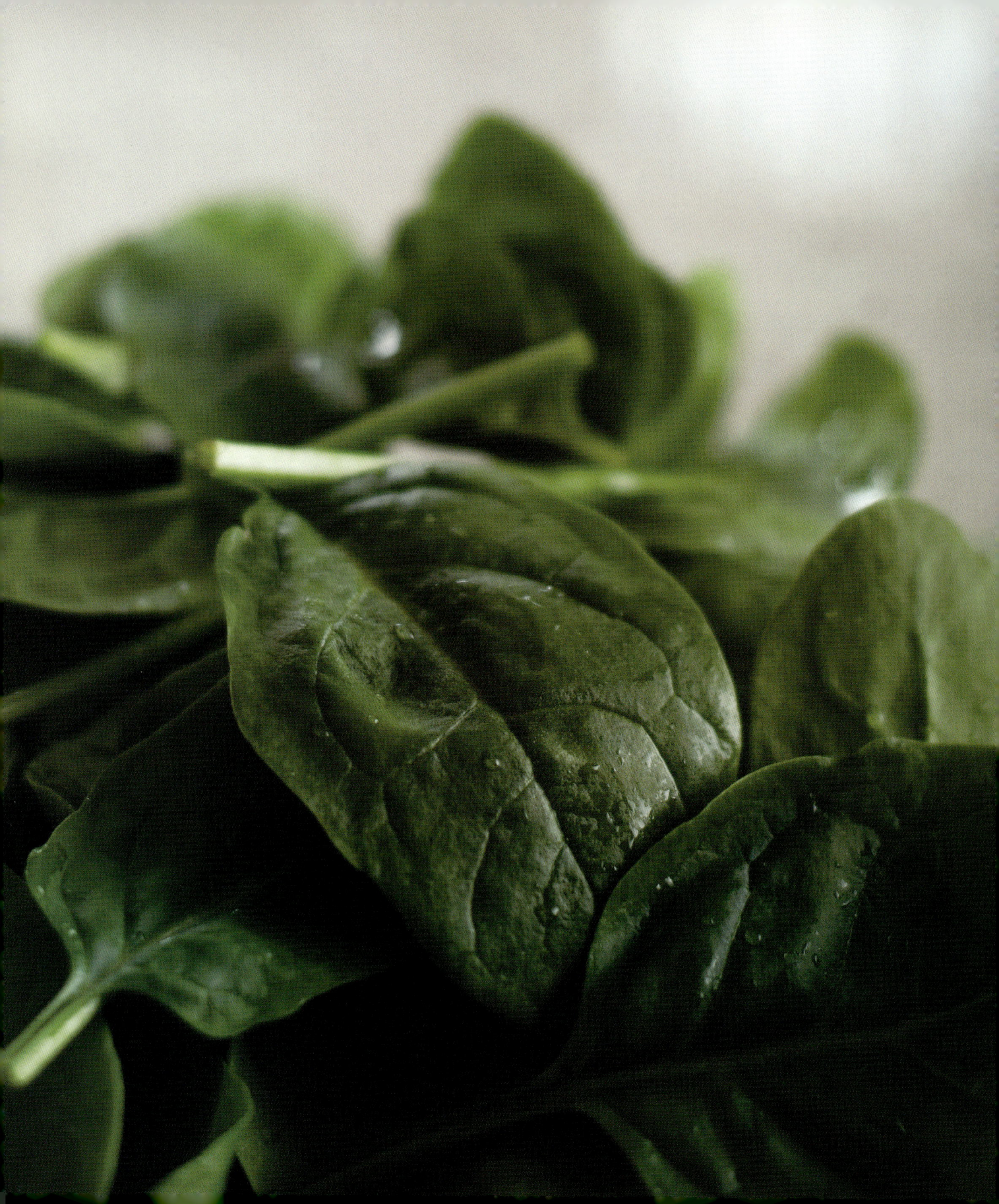

Food for your lifestyle

This chapter will help you devise a solid plan to achieve your best lifestyle and optimal health. And, of course, whip that body back into shape! You can overcome obstacles to a healthy diet with organisation, planning, time management, creativity and just a little compromise. A good attitude doesn't hurt either.

The last chapter covered the *what* and *why* of food. This one discusses *how* and *when* to eat positively with a couple of toddlers and a newborn under your wing. Your lifestyle is dynamic and your nutrition must be flexible enough to adapt for different requirements as your circumstances change—through pregnancies, breastfeeding, toddler years and beyond.

So follow the steps in this chapter and give yourself the gift of health, which no-one else can give you. Consider 'diet' in its positive sense and your healthy life starts now.

THE FOOD DIARY

The first step to improving your nutrition is to work out what you're currently eating. You may think you know what you eat, but the proof is in the food diary. Many women say they hardly eat a thing and still can't lose weight—but they usually eat more than they realise. They restrict their food at mealtimes, only to overcompensate by grazing all day and night! A food diary accurately shows areas for improvement, so you can tweak your eating habits to work *for* you, not *against* you.

This is not an exhaustive kilojoule-counting assignment; it is very easy. All you need is some paper and a pen. Put them in a handy location, like the kitchen, and write down everything you eat and drink for seven days.

Ready?

Find out what you're really eating

Improve your diet today

Set up your environment for success

Easy ideas for meals, snacks and healthy cooking

The lowdown on 'low-fat' and 'light' food

Feeding little people and big people without a fuss

Get your plan together and swing into action

- Quantities do not need to be measured or weighed. Just estimate, for example 1/2 cup, 3 scoops, 2 slices.
- Just eat normally—don't try to be 'good'. You need a true representation of your eating quality, quantity and patterns and your current lifestyle.
- If you have a meal out or takeaway, include it on your list with an accurate description of what you eat. It is sometimes difficult to know exactly what is in a curry or takeaway pizza. Just list the dish with the main ingredients. For example: Indian curry—1 cup lamb, potatoes, peas, curry sauce plus 1 cup rice; or Hawaiian pizza—3 slices ($\frac{1}{3}$ of family size), bread base, cheese, pineapple, ham, tomato sauce.
- Don't forget the nibbles. Note even a handful of nuts, or finishing your toddler's sandwich crusts.

You may or may not be surprised by this record, but it is an important reference from which to start. The best diet for you works not only for you, but also for your family and lifestyle. It is the one you can sustain with least resistance and maximum benefit.

The results

After seven days, sit down and take a good look at what you ate over the week. Compare it to the following checklist of optimal eating strategies.

- Eight glasses of water a day, or at least six with other non-caffeinated drinks.
- A larger quantity of food eaten earlier in the day. For example, if you're awake from 6 a.m. until 10 p.m., more food should be eaten in the first half of your day (by 2 p.m.) than in the second half.
- Do you eat according to a fairly regular schedule? Ideally your three main meals will be fairly evenly spread, with two snacks in between. Eating lunch two hours late or skipping breakfast altogether will often cause you to overeat in compensation and make poorer food choices, e.g. fast food.
- Quality of food—preferably mostly home-prepared or cooked from fresh ingredients. Minimal processed food.
- No more than one takeaway dinner a week. Preferably not high in fat, salt or sugar (it does exist!).

- No more than two cups of caffeinated drinks a day (coffee, tea).
- Junk food: as little as possible, as it only works against you. Sensible allowances for a little 'soul food' here and there.
- Check your diary against the food pyramid detailed in chapter 5. Are you eating mostly vegetables, dried peas, beans, lentils, cereals, bread, fruit and nuts? Are you eating lean meat, eggs, fish, chicken (skinless), milk, yoghurt and cheese moderately? Are you eating these in small amounts: oil, margarine, reduced-fat spreads, butter and sugar? Or is your pyramid lopsided or upside down?
- Crosscheck your diary against the recommended servings in chapter 5. A serving is, for example, a slice of bread, a piece of fruit or a glass of milk. A quick way to gauge an appropriate amount of daily protein for you is a piece of meat (or substitute) the size and thickness of your palm. Also pay attention to the *relative proportions* as these are designed to ensure a balanced intake of essential nutrients, including vitamins and minerals. Don't worry if the balance isn't ideal every day. If it more or less evens out over the week, you're doing all right. If you notice an obvious deficiency in a particular group, add more of this instead of another group you're eating in excess.
- If you're sure your portions are reasonable and you exercise but can't lose weight, examine the *quality* of your food choices. Increase fibrous, filling starches (fruits, vegies, whole grains) and lean protein, decrease fat, alcohol and sugars and you will cut kilojoules without eating any less!
- Determine if you eat on autopilot. Do you eat at certain times or places, whether hungry or not? For example, picking while cooking, grazing between meals, or snacking in the car. Other dangerous habits include 'upsizing' your meal because it's better value, finishing your plate because it's there, eating when you're tired, bored or upset, and drinking alcohol daily. These little things add up to blow your energy intake sky-high without you noticing.

After the food diary exercise you will have a good idea which areas need improving and which habits are working against you.

Write a list of the things you need to alter in your diet. Start with the most obvious: for example, if you're drinking five cola drinks and only one glass of water a day. Add the smaller, more subtle changes you require: perhaps you get two serves of fruit only sometimes, not every day.

Then start making changes with the first item on your list. Make modifications at a level you feel comfortable with. Positive eating is focusing on 'what is the best thing I can eat now'. Be realistic—too little change and you're not helping; too much and you'll feel deprived and relapse to old ways. Try substituting or reducing portions of less positive foods rather than cutting them out altogether. Changing habits in smaller steps helps you adjust and you'll barely notice or miss anything, particularly if you add a positive food or habit for every less optimal one you subtract. As soon as you adapt to one small change, try a couple more. Before you know it, your body will start reaping the rewards.

PURGE THE PANTRY

And the fridge and the freezer and your shopping list. Chapter 5 listed some foods you shouldn't stock regularly as they impede your fitness goals. Remember, you *can* include special indulgences, but no-one needs a constant supply of chips, sweets, cakes, chocolates and soft drinks at home. They are no good for children either, so the sooner you find better alternatives the better. Children are happy with 100 per cent dried fruit straps, air-popped popcorn, pretzels, yoghurt, muffins sweetened with fruit or rice crackers if that's what they get used to. They learn what a 'treat' and a snack is from you; choose wisely for them.

Now it's time to organise your food so good nutrition just happens to you . . .

The following lists of basic items to stock in your home are simply an example or a starting point. Keep these ingredients on hand so you'll always be able to rustle up a quick, healthy meal or snack without too much effort, and won't resort to fast food. Alter them to suit your own tastes and preferences. Some items are less ideal than others, but score big points for convenience, without being exactly *un*healthy. No-one's perfect all the time, and a less-than-ideal option is still better than giving up altogether!

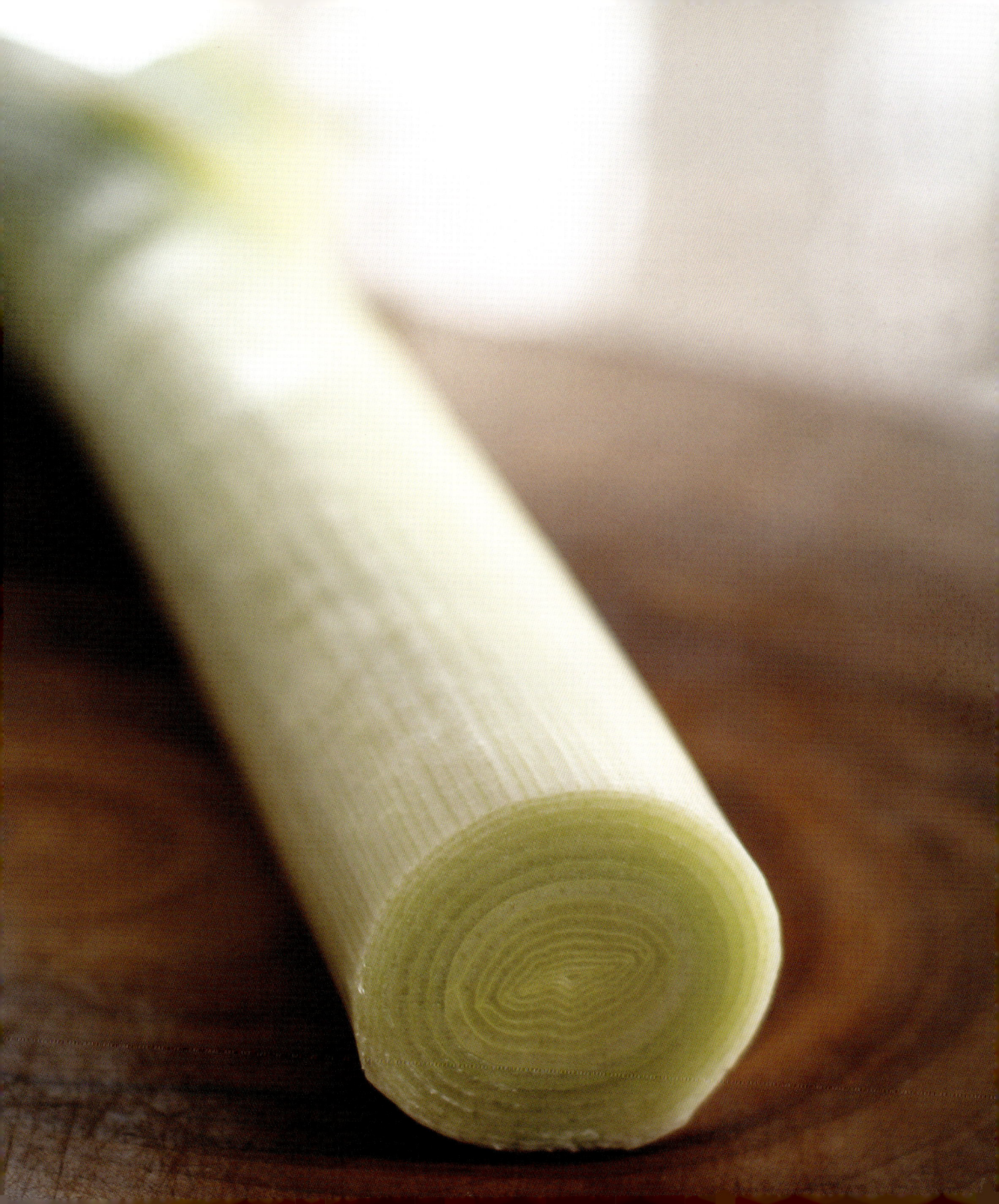

Pantry

BAKING NEEDS
- Wholemeal, plain and self-raising flour, rice flour, cornflour, almond meal etc.
- Sugar (you'll need *some*): brown, white or raw and caster sugar

PASTA, RICE, PULSES
- A variety of pasta shapes and flavours: spaghetti, fettuccine, penne, spinach or wholemeal etc.
- Rice: arborio (for risotto), basmati rice (provides longer-lasting energy than jasmine rice), dried rice noodles
- Dried legumes (pulses), such as lentils, split peas, chickpeas and beans like red kidney, butter and canelli.

CEREALS, GRAINS
- Choose those low in refined sugar and added fats and colours: rolled oats/porridge, semolina, quinoa, couscous, multi-grain cereals, mixes with added fruits, nuts and fibre
- Packaged tortillas or naan breads: they're preserved, but long-lasting and very handy

CANNED/TETRA-PACKED FOOD
- Vegetables and fruit: chopped tomatoes, sun-dried tomatoes, creamed corn, beans (pinto, kidney, baked etc.), artichokes, olives, capers, pickles, fruits in natural juice with no added sugar
- Seafood: tuna, salmon, sardines, oysters
- Juice: 100% fruit juice (no added sugar), passionfruit pulp etc.
- Soup: vegetable, chicken, mushroom etc. Look for natural ingredients and low salt (sodium)
- Other: canned spaghetti (a good snack, but watch the sodium)

COOKING NEEDS/CONDIMENTS
- Tomato paste, quality pasta sauces
- Oil: Plant oils such as olive, canola, sunflower, hazelnut and sesame.
- Vinegar: white and balsamic
- Mustard (Dijon, American, English), cranberry sauce, chutney, mayonnaise (light if you like), vinaigrette, salad dressing (light)
- Spreads: Vegemite, honey, peanut butter, 100% fruit jam

- Sauces and marinades: soy sauce, Worcestershire, tomato, BBQ, teriyaki, spicy plum, satay, honey soy, black bean, hoi sin. Look for ones with natural ingredients, low sodium and sugar
- Quality cooking stock (if you find time, make your own)
- Dried herbs and spices—the full collection, and learn how to use them

OTHER FOODS

- Dried fruit, nuts—look for fewer preservatives like sulfur dioxide (preservative 220)
- Rice crackers—read the labels here as some brands are no better than chips. Watch out for artificial colours and flavours, excessive sodium and added fat
- Water crackers, pretzels and plain popcorn to pop at home

Freezer

- Dinner shortcuts: plain pizza bases, lasagne (low in fat, made with natural ingredients), snap-frozen seafood (tastes very fresh), home-cooked or bought meals (casseroles, curries)
- Frozen vegetables: peas, carrots, corn, chopped onions, stir-fry mixes, oven-bake potato chips
- Frozen cake for a morning tea drop-in

Fridge

DAIRY

- Cheese: cottage, ricotta, cream, tasty, mould/soft, parmesan—reduced-fat versions if you like
- Milk: full cream for the kids and light/skim for you
- Butter, margarine or a healthier substitute like olive oil spread
- Low-fat yoghurt sweetened with fruit (no added sugar or artificial sweetener)

PRODUCE

- Fresh, seasonal fruits, vegetables and herbs to inspire your meals

OTHER FOODS

- Eggs, short-cut bacon, non-processed lunch meats (ham off the bone), turkey breast, lean cuts of meat and poultry, fish, smoked fish, other seafood
- Fresh noodles, pasta, tofu

HITTING THE SHOPS

Someone has to be in charge of hunting and gathering, but you don't have to physically do it all yourself. Having fresh food magically arrive in the first months with a new baby makes a huge difference. A couple of my friends successfully offloaded the food shopping to their husbands on a permanent basis. Well done, girls! For the rest of us, at least get him to pick up the milk and fresh bread during the week. You make the list and hand it on—delegate.

When my children were newborns I used online shopping for larger items and dry goods (nappies, toilet paper, laundry powder, soap, pantry items), but I always preferred to choose the fresh produce, seafood and meat myself. If you don't have access to online shopping, many shops home-deliver to a local area—ask around. You can fax or phone an order and delivery fees are usually minimal or free if it's close.

Shop without the entourage if possible. There's nothing worse than being at the checkout with the screaming baby and escaping toddler, getting looks ranging from pity to severe annoyance, but no help. Try shopping alone on nights or weekends when your partner is with the children. You can concentrate, relax and even stop for a coffee.

If you must take the children, keep as many strapped in as possible. Combinations of baby pouches, prams and trolley seats will expedite the trip. Next, anaesthetise them with healthy snacks or portable activities or toys. Shopping bores little people quickly and they will find 'other ways' to stay amused—which I guarantee will not amuse you, or the shopkeeper. Older children can help put things in the trolley and hold the list. Have a list prepared so you can get in and out faster without pondering.

If you plan meals and write lists, you can shop just once a week. It's easy to cover seven days, or at least get the week done and be flexible on weekends. You may need bread more frequently, but quality produce will get you through the week. For example, use more perishable foods such as lettuce, celery, cabbage, spinach, berries and cut melons earlier in the week. Other foods such as avocado, stone fruit, bananas, apples, pears, citrus, cucumbers, tomatoes, eggplant and zucchini should easily last a week if fresh. Buy enough meat for the week, refrigerate some for a few days and freeze the rest. Eggs and dairy usually last longer than a week—check the use-by dates.

Don't shop for food when you're hungry; you'll buy more and make poorer choices. When you're hungry, everything looks good! Stick to your list and don't buy on impulse, unless something you buy every week is on special, in which case stock up.

Having a meal plan for the week can guide your choices for produce and meats, but stay flexible to allow for the freshest seasonal and best-priced food. Look for inspiration in recipe magazines or cookbooks. Regularly trying a new ingredient will help you expand your repertoire, and you might find some new family favourites.

MEAL INSPIRATION

Here are some ideas for meals and snacks, to which you can add. Most are focussed on being healthy, but some compromise a little to make life easier. Remember, you need more energy earlier in the day. Dinner is often the largest (and sometimes the only 'proper') meal, in which we try to squeeze all the day's vegetables and protein. Try to distribute these nutrients into lunches, breakfasts and snacks as well.

A meal does not have to be 'cuisine'; it can just be food! Some of the quick dinner suggestions—including my favourite: breakfast for dinner!—save your sanity when food is the last thing on your mind.

Breakfast

The 'queen's meal'. You will use most energy from this meal, as opposed to storing it, and it will kickstart your metabolism for the day. Breakfast like the Japanese, who may have green tea, steamed rice, miso soup with tofu, grilled fish, omelette, eggs or vegetables. Most Westerners would consider this a dinner meal, but we're the ones who have it all wrong! A muffin and coffee or bowl of sugared flakes won't get you far if your day involves breastfeeding, kindy-gym, work and exercise.

If you feel you can't eat in the morning, start with a glass of water, or something dry like toast rather than coffee or juice, to dilute stomach acid that may have concentrated due to having fasted and dehydrated overnight—morning sickness taught me this one. Get out the breakfast dishes and cereal boxes the night before, plan what to have and get up early enough to eat without rushing.

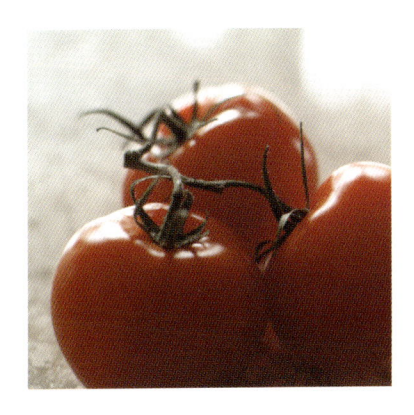

It's easy to get in a breakfast rut. Not being much of a morning person myself, I know inspiration is slow on rising. Make a list, keep it in the kitchen and add to it any time you think of something new. I came across a great website with over 1500 breakfast recipes: www.mrbreakfast.com. It has sections for healthy breakfasts, international breakfasts, brunches and fun ideas for children. If you can't find something there, you're not trying!

Porridge is the breakfast of champions. Other cereals are also a great and easy way to get long-lasting energy from starch and fibre, if you pick the right one. Look for low *added* fat, low sugar, high fibre, more whole grains and less processing—it's all on the label. 'Diet' or 'light' cereals are often so processed and airy they don't get you through the next hour, let alone to the next meal. Cereals mixed with fruits and nuts are great (they will have a little more natural fat from the nuts), but be careful with toasted muesli, which can be very high in added fat. Try adding low-fat yoghurt or fruit to increase the palatability of blander but very healthy cereals. Do I need to even mention that sugary, coloured or chocolate cereals should not even make it to the checkout, let alone the breakfast table? Remember, you determine your children's habits—lead by example and have a healthy start to your day.

Fat: if you really want the bacon, the pastry or the butter on toast, have it for breakfast, as you have the *potential* to burn it off if you're active. It's better than trying to be 'good' all day and then giving in to the Danish pastry late at night. Don't go overboard though, and do find a way to use up the energy or you *will* store it.

Eggs are a quick and nutritious source of quality protein. The only fat is in the yolk, so you can just eat the whites if you're concerned. But I wouldn't bother. In comparison to the fat added to popular packaged and processed foods, the amount of fat in a few eggs is negligible. Scrambled eggs on wholegrain toast, with a side of fruit and trimmed bacon, gets all engines firing and stops you overcompensating later. If time is tight in the morning, boil some eggs the night before, refrigerate and then reheat.

Wholegrain toast or toasted sandwiches are great, but don't just have the same old 'breakfast' spreads like jam or Vegemite. Get into 'lunch foods' like ham, cheese and tomato, creamed corn, baked beans, smoked salmon and cottage or cream cheese for a satisfying meal. Watch out for fatty spreads like butter—you really don't need it unless a filling is very dry. Try going without; you may be surprised how quickly tastes adapt.

Fruit is packed with vitamins, fibre and carbohydrate energy, so you can have as much as you want for breakfast. Make a mixed fruit salad the night before and top it with low-fat yoghurt and a handful of grainy cereal—delicious! Stewed or puréed fruits (especially berries), fruit juice or passionfruit pulp make great 'dressings' for fruit salad. If you're running late, at least grab a banana and a box of sultanas on your way out as they are much better choices than most 'breakfast bars', which are embarrassingly high in sugar and low in quality starches.

A breakfast smoothie will keep you going if you add the right ingredients: low-fat yoghurt, 100 per cent fruit juice, a scoop of wheat bran, a banana and other fruits. (Beware of takeaway smoothies, which are often high in fat.) These are also good for an occasional quick snack, but watch the portion size and frequency—they are high in energy and you can drink faster than you can eat!

Lunch

Try to get some protein, fruit and vegetables at lunch. Lunch is one of the main meals, and if you can't stomach a big breakfast, then have a decent lunch.

So long as you have some bread and something to put on it there's always the humble sandwich. However, one sandwich with a simple spread like honey just isn't sufficient for lunch, even when trying to lose weight. Make your sandwiches on 'meaty' breads like wholegrain or rye. White bread is junk food—'sometimes' food; it's processed too quickly by the body and doesn't give enough nutrition for the amount of calories it provides. There's no need to give white bread to children either—remember they eat what they get used to from an early age.

To get more flavour with fewer kilojoules, substitute butter with lower-fat dressings and spreads such as mustard, chutney, fat-reduced mayonnaise, salsa or cranberry sauce. Add salad leaves, herbs, sprouts, turkey, ham, salmon, tuna, boiled or scrambled egg, roast meat, chicken, rocket, tomato, cheese . . . the list goes on. Think of healthy, delicious options, keeping it as fresh as possible (minimal processing) and low in fat. If you really need some fat on your bread, use a scraping of canola, olive or vegetable-oil margarine for a healthier heart.

Have dinner for lunch. The meat-and-three-veg routine is better suited to this time of the day. Our European friends can teach us much about stopping for a gastronomic event every day (followed by a nap). Left-overs are great for lunch, so cook extra, or eat less for dinner and finish it for lunch the next day. If you work, take lunch as often as possible, as it's kinder on your body and wallet. Just remember to throw in an ice-pack if you can't refrigerate. If you must get takeaway, find a sandwich bar where you can get something fresh.

Dinner

This is the meal which requires more effort and planning because we seem to feel dinner should be different or more interesting. But don't convince yourself you need a major culinary production at night—food is just fine. Shortly after dinner your metabolic rate slows to resting, and you don't need much energy to sustain basic body functions. If you exercise or are active during the day, you need energy to refuel and repair muscles. If you want to lose weight, don't overcompensate for your exercise by 'rewarding' with food. Remember, you don't earn food or kilojoules; you eat first pay later.

Start a list of dinner ideas as you read this section, then tackle that pile of dusty cookbooks and magazines and add to your list. Ask friends for their favourite meal ideas, and remember there's a world full of suggestions online.

If you really want to run a tight ship, allocate a couple of nights for set meals, such as Friday night barbecue (Dad cooks!), Wednesday night pasta or vegetarian and Sunday night roast. I like Saturday night home-made pizza and movie night. Then to fill the other few nights, slot in whatever you buy fresh that week, no recipes required, such as a simple cut of marinated meat, grilled chicken or steamed fish and vegies.

If you exercise at night, have a larger breakfast and lunch. Eat a small early dinner, then after the session, drink water and eat a small snack to replace energy in the blood and muscles, but don't go overboard. Have a warm shower, relax with herbal tea or stretches and go to bed. However, beware of eating so early that you graze at the fridge later.

Freezer cooking is essential for new mums. In the early days with a baby, you may be lucky enough to have people who bring you meals for the freezer. Pay attention to what they bring. When compiling your list of meal ideas, mark the ones which freeze well, then cook double quantities of these every time. When you get into a routine, this gives you at least one night off a week and you still get healthy home-cooked meals.

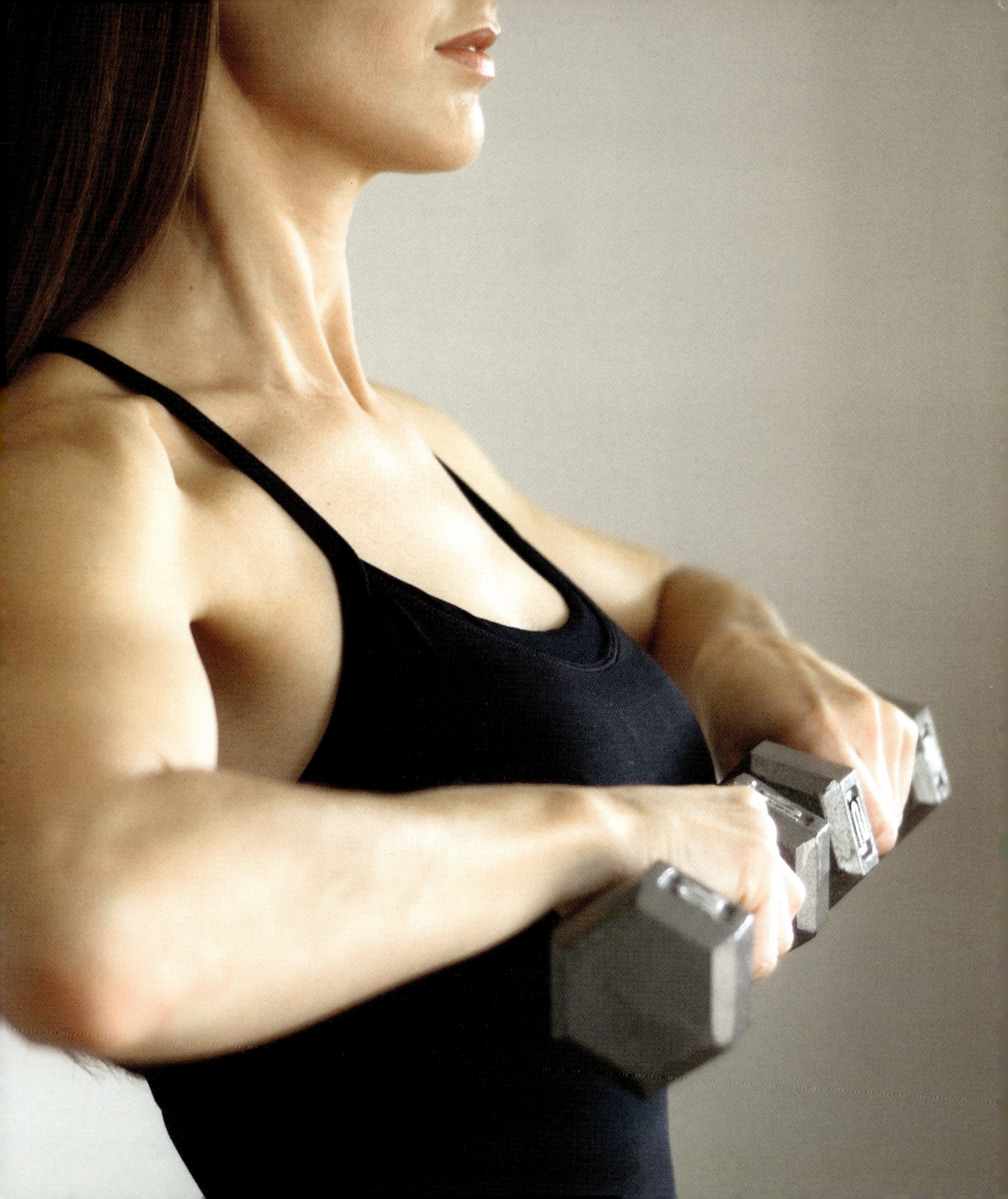

'Healthy' takeaway does exist! We all need a break sometimes, especially on days when nothing goes to plan. As long as it's not every day and you choose reasonably healthy options, it's fine to have takeaway as a meal option. For example, buy a barbecued chicken (skip the skin) and supplement it with fresh salad at home. A favourite of ours is takeaway Thai ginger prawns eaten at home with steamed rice and vegetables, which is easier than eating in the restaurant with small children anyway. One of my regular 'stand-by' meals is from a local pasta shop. I get a couple of dishes of mixed pasta and salad. I usually choose vegetarian dishes and tomato-based over cream sauces and my children love it! When choosing pasta, avoid getting varieties with both meat and cheese, to keep the saturated fat down.

I also keep a frozen lasagne as a shortcut. I've found one which has fresh ingredients, is lower in fat than others and tastes good. My local deli stocks fresh, locally made pre-packed meals which can be frozen and are good for 'Plan B' nights. Examine your local options. Get menus from nearby takeaway restaurants and make a list of the healthier options for when you run out of food or declare you're not cooking tonight—which every mum has the right to do!

Local pizza shops usually offer a good-quality product compared with the large chains. They are usually wood-fired, often 'gourmet', smaller and more expensive—but if they're healthy and they deliver, it's worth it. We can get a quality pizza from the 'change bowl' in the kitchen—the coins men refuse to carry in their pockets and collect daily. Our local pizzerias offer thinner crusts with plenty of fresh topping options, and they're generally better than I could cook at home. Choose pizzas with vegetables and interesting sauces and herbs instead of processed meats or lots of cheese.

Other dishes dripping with hidden fat and kilojoules are those delicious, creamy Indian and Thai curries. For Indian, choose meats cooked in the tandoor and lighter vegetarian dishes. For Thai and Chinese food, choose stir-fried meals with lots of vegetables cooked in sauces such as soy, oyster, chilli, garlic and ginger, with fragrant herbs like basil and lemongrass. Stay away from deep-fried appetisers and ice cream. Most traditional Japanese food is healthy—especially sushi—but watch the volume of food if you have teppanyaki (Japanese barbecue).

Fast food such as burgers, fries, pizzas and fried chicken are 'sometimes' food at most, as they are high in fat, salt, kilojoules and preservatives and are too highly processed to form a regular part of a healthy diet.

Breakfast for dinner happens on weekends at my house. This is such a simple solution. You generally have 'breakfast' foods in the house—but who says they can only be eaten in the morning? Scrambled eggs, toast, baked beans, omelettes, yoghurt and fruit provide many a balanced dinner that my kids enjoy. Even cereal, trimmed bacon and home-made pancakes with tinned fruit are faster and healthier options than a drive-through burger and fries. Omelettes are particularly versatile, with the fillings limited only by your imagination and what's in the fridge: cheese and pineapple, sliced mushrooms, grated zucchini, canned spaghetti, tomato and herbs, corn, ricotta, spinach . . .

Consider having one or two vegetarian meals for dinner each week, as you can get ample protein from legumes, whole grains, nuts, eggs, dairy and vegetables. If you have a good serve of meat for lunch, there's no need to have it at dinner as well.

Fish is fantastically healthy and even the oilier varieties are so good for you. Fish is delicious marinated and barbecued or steamed with lemon and herbs. There are so many varieties, including some less 'fishy' options like fresh swordfish and tuna. Large deep-sea fish contain higher trace amounts of mercury, so if you're pregnant or breastfeeding, limit seafood intake to two to three serves per week of any fish or seafood, except for the fish listed below:

- limit orange roughy (deep sea perch) or catfish to one serve per week, with no other fish that week or
- limit shark (also called flake, which is often used in takeaway fish and chips, so ask what you're eating) or billfish (broadbill, swordfish and marlin) to one serve per fortnight, with no other fish that fortnight.

More information can be found at the New South Wales government's Food Authority website at www.foodauthority.nsw.gov.au.

Snacks

Mid-morning and mid-afternoon snacks keep your energy high and blood nutrient levels stable. They also stop you arriving totally famished at meals and overeating. If you keep main meal portions modest and snacks small, five meals a day can actually total less food than three huge meals when you're starving. Eating several smaller meals also keeps your metabolic rate buzzing along as your body uses energy to process the food and uses readily available fuel for energy demands. If you have three large meals each day—or more commonly, a pitiful breakfast if any, a little lunch and a huge dinner—your body is taught to process and store energy for those long hours without. But this is not a suggestion to graze all day. Morning and afternoon snacks need to be consciously planned so you're satisfied without adding to your waistline.

When you go out, you probably take snacks for your children, so take a healthy snack for yourself as well. This ensures you don't skip meals (a big no-no for weight control) and prevents you foraging for a high-sugar hit while out. The easiest thing to take is fruit, like a banana, mandarin or apple. I also use small plastic containers and zip-lock bags for snacks like pretzels, plain popcorn, rice crackers, grapes, strawberries, chopped fruit, sultanas, breakfast cereal, little pikelets or corn cakes and chopped cucumber, celery or carrot. Although they are higher in sugar and fat, I always have a couple of fruit muesli bars at the bottom of my bag, as they're still better than doughnuts.

When you're at home, make snacks more interesting, like a small lunch. A small sandwich, a fruit salad, a tub of yoghurt, crackers and cheese, vegetables with salsa, and breakfast cereal are just some ideas. Keep it fresh, healthy and a small serving size—something which fits easily on a bread plate, not a dinner plate.

LOW-FAT, 'LIGHT' AND DIET FOODS

There are plenty of naturally grown foods which are low in fat or kilojoules. They don't come with labels and are the ones to eat most often. However, when it comes to packaged food, never rely on terms such as 'lite', 'light', 'low-fat', 'diet', 'low-carb' and 'low-GI'—always read the nutrition panel and ingredients list. Some of these products are so artificial that you're better off just having a smaller amount of the full-fat

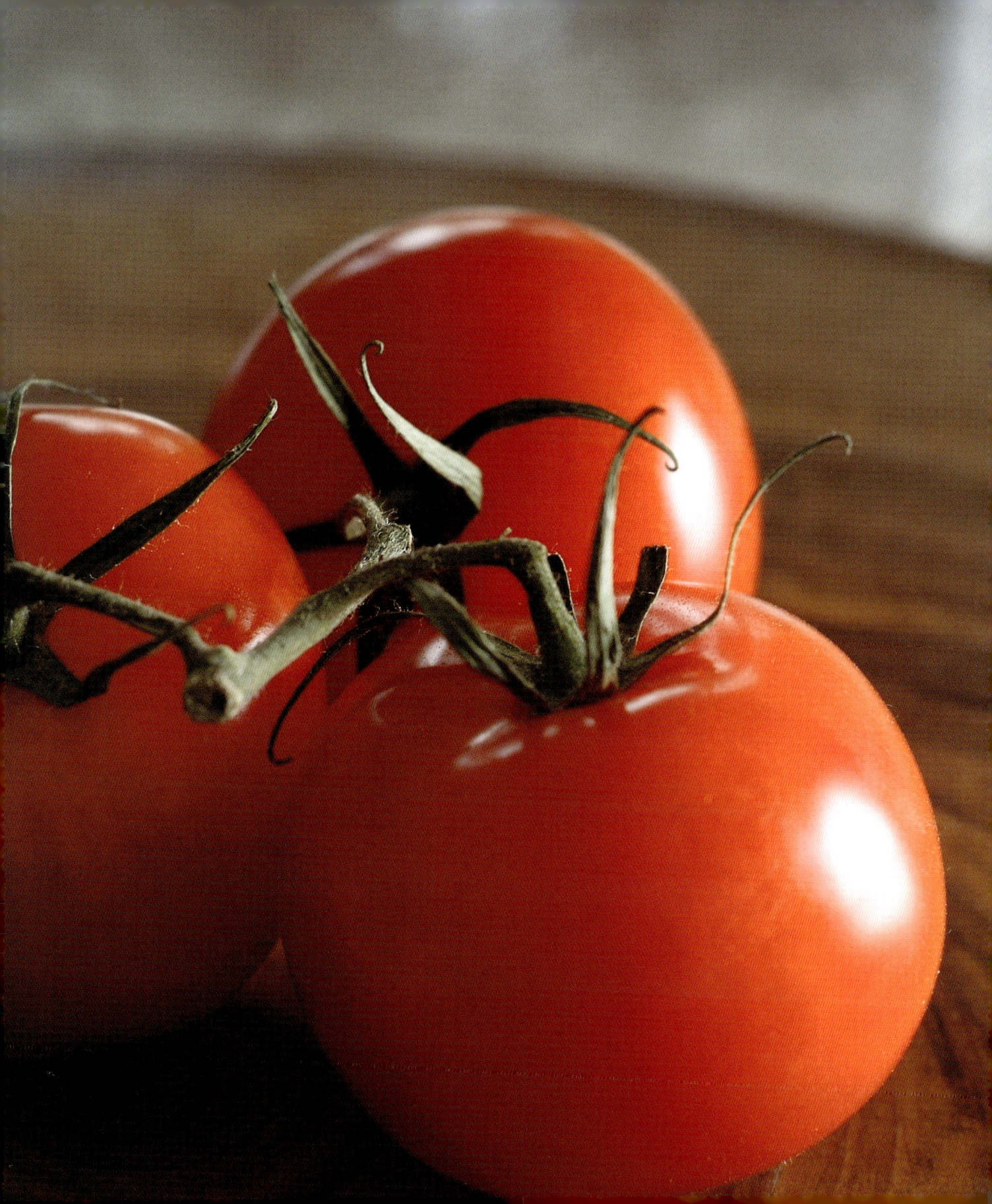

or natural version. The term 'light' can also mean light in flavour, texture, colour or consistency (as in olive oil for example), not always kilojoules, so read carefully.

I don't recommend artificial sweeteners, firstly because they're artificial and secondly because they seem to work more on the mind than body. I wonder at people who carry a personal supply of artificial sweetener to have in their coffee, yet have a muffin as well or a soft drink later, both of which have mountains of sugar. One teaspoon of sweetener or sugar in a coffee is so negligible compared to most other sources of refined sugar, and too often it justifies eating more kilojoules because you're having a 'diet' drink.

Look out for artificial sweeteners in diet yoghurts and ice cream as well and go for brands sweetened with added fruit instead.

Infants and toddlers should never eat low-fat, diet or light foods or milk unless specifically recommended by a doctor.

'MY KIDS WON'T EAT THAT!'

Don't let fussy eaters condition you to cook especially for them. This will only reinforce their picky habits, and worsen as they get older. It's vital to introduce young children to a wide variety of foods and flavours to ensure a well-balanced and colourful diet and to set them up for a life of good nutrition. Anyone with a toddler knows there are several reasons they may not eat something: it could be too green, too puffy, too hot or too cold, too ugly, too funny, too big, too small, too mushy, too stringy or just 'yuk'. The only way to deal with picky eaters is to never give in, ever. I know; I was one and I have one.

Try foods repeatedly, in small quantities and in different ways, different shapes and different textures (cooked, raw, chopped or mashed). It's all about disguise, presentation, promotion and distraction. Also, getting children involved in food preparation can increase their enthusiasm when it's time to eat. Let them help and teach them skills appropriate to their age. Cooking is an invaluable life skill.

In terms of easy meals for all the family, start out how you intend to continue. If you want to offer four different meals every night—one for babies, one for little children, one for you and one for the man—you'd better open a restaurant and get paid as it will be a full-time job. Never force-feed, but don't accept children knocking back food on instinct, as allowing is reinforcing. Learn to adapt meals for different eating stages, such as puréeing for baby or leaving spicy sauces off until last to keep it child-friendly. This means less time in the kitchen for you!

INTO THE KITCHEN

I'm not the world's best cook. I'm a good cook: I can follow a recipe, I can adapt, improvise, substitute, prepare most common foods and throw a simple brunch or barbecue. But above all I am a healthy cook. No-one will get heart disease from my food. That's not to say there's no fat, salt, flavour or texture in what I prepare. But I just concentrate on keeping things as fresh and varied as possible.

I approach the challenge of 'healthifying' recipes as a research scientist and have found that success lies in moderation, never the extremes. For example, if you take all the sugar out of a muffin recipe, it won't taste much better than plain toast. Then if you also omit all the fat, it's plain *dry* toast. I simply look for healthier alternatives, which add flavour, texture, taste, fibre, vitamins, minerals and essential fats. Fruits and fruit purées are the easiest way to add sweetness. Of course fruit sugars also contain kilojoules, but you get the vitamins and you can use less than normal sugar, as you get the marvellous fruit flavour as well. Many fruits also make muffins and cakes juicy and reduce the amount of fat needed—mashed banana and puréed apple, mango, apricot, pear or berries all work well. Chunks of fruit, nuts and even chocolate chips (yes, chocolate chips!) are great for texture and taste. Consider this: if you make chocolate-chip muffins using a commercial muffin mix or conventional recipe it is loaded with sugar and fat. If you take most of that out, add back a few chocolate chips or sultanas and some mashed banana and wholemeal flour, you've got something you could eat daily as part of a balanced diet which tastes almost too good to be true!

When you use recipes, don't be afraid to change the ingredients. If a recipe calls for oil, butter or cream, consider options to substitute—for example, milk, juice, a purée, soup, stock, wine, water, yoghurt, sour cream etc. Or let go of recipes altogether and experiment, re-create, use variety and reap the rewards in terms of health and enjoyment of food.

PULLING IT ALL TOGETHER

You're the managing director, so run your life like every good business: with a plan. Prepare, organise, delegate, execute. Now that you have all the tools, get out your weekly schedule. Find time slots for your shopping, cooking and meal planning. Write your meal plan for the next week and put it somewhere handy. Once you get into a routine this takes less time than foraging for takeaway every second night. When you get half an hour to relax on the weekend, flip through magazines and add to your meal ideas. Your collection will grow and you'll get used to planning as the weeks roll on.

When I had little babies, my dinner schedule worked as follows.

Sunday: peruse meal ideas over late breakfast and shop by myself for the week. Dinner was something fresh, like seafood, often barbecued.

Monday: freezer cooking—make double quantity. Chop and prepare ingredients during baby's morning nap. Put the food on early if it's a casserole and let it cook.

Tuesday: no cooking today. Freezer meal from Monday last week.

Wednesday: cook a quick noodle, pasta or stir-fry dish.

Thursday: defrost meat or chicken (bought Sunday) for a meat-and-veg meal.

Friday: takeaway (healthy).

Saturday: home-made pizza, or Dad's night to cook.

Broken down like this, it's relatively simple. You may be doing something like this already without realising it. Having your food on autopilot means you don't have to be organised every day. Your life will be easier and healthier.

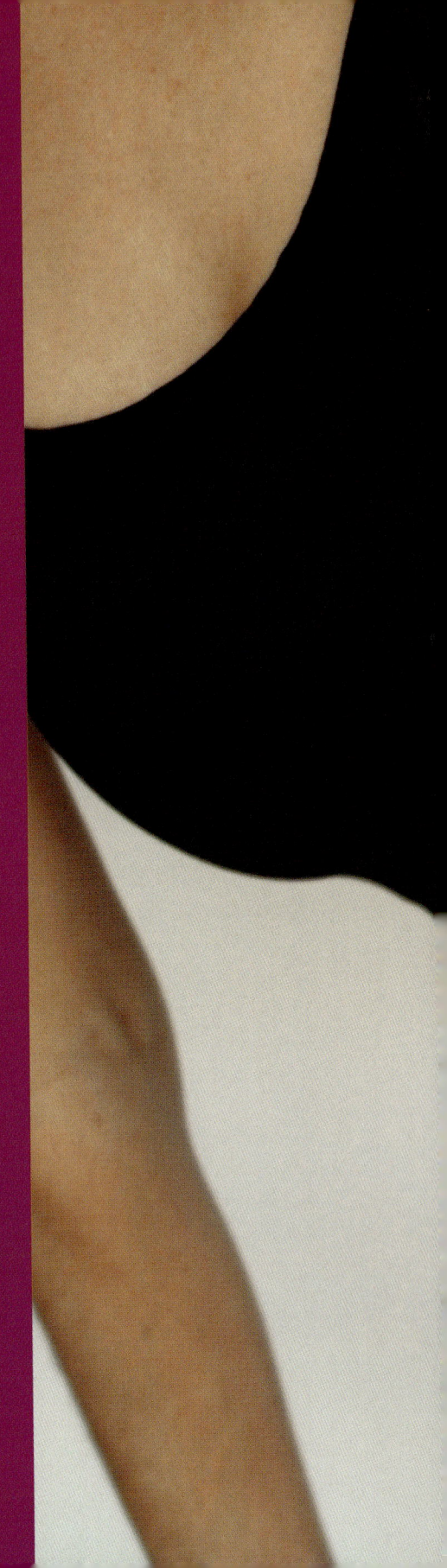

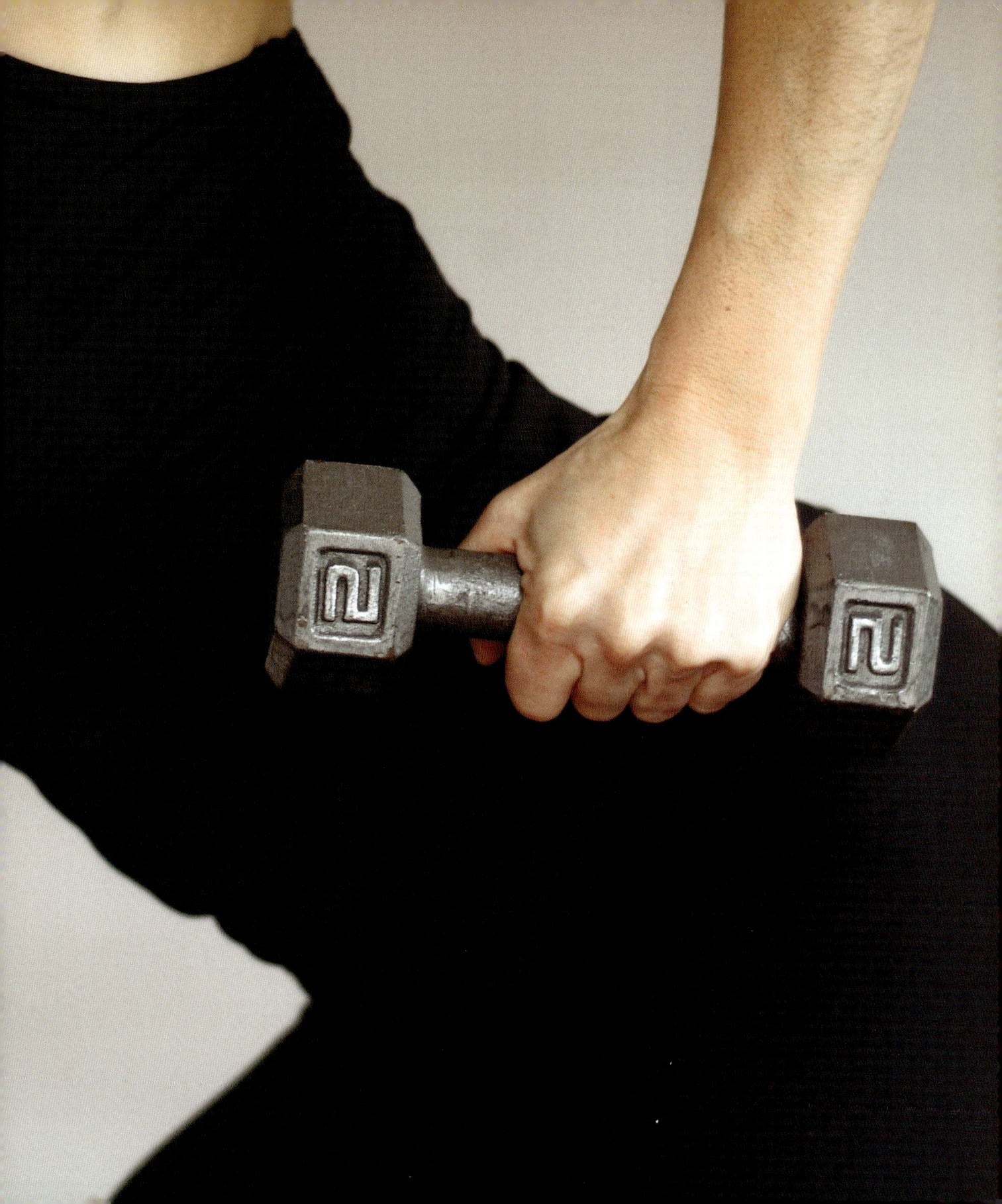

Action

Do the food diary exercise

Examine current food habits and write a list of improvements

Fill your kitchen and shopping lists with fresh food for positive eating

Eat smaller and more frequent meals

Collect and organise recipes you like for easy reference

Prioritise getting and preparing fresh food in your weekly schedule

Case study: Sam

I worked on an exercise and nutrition program for my friend Sam, who has two toddlers. Sam had a few kilos to lose, was unfit, tired and wanted to get back in shape. She was on the children's eating schedule all day, until it came to their dinner at about 6 p.m., which she skipped, waiting for her husband to return from work around 7.30 p.m. Then one of them cooked—often her husband—or they frequently had takeaway. They didn't eat until 8.30 p.m. So there were two separate dinners every night—one for the kids, one for the grown-ups.

Sam said she was very irritable from the children's dinnertime until hers, and attributed this to doing the whole dinner-bath-bed routine alone after a long day with tired little ones—taxing on every mum! Sam's food diary revealed she was rushing a quick bite for breakfast and lunch, but dinner was the one meal for which she relaxed and ate most of her energy and nutrients.

I immediately suggested planning meals so the family could have just one meal each evening, even if it was eaten in 'shifts'. Preparing entirely separate meals for the two 'dinner shifts' is just too much work; most of us don't feel like cooking the first meal, let alone a second! Most meals reheat well but items which don't—like grilled fish or steak—can be prepared just before serving, with everything else on standby.

I also suggested Sam eat with her children during the week. It's lovely for her and her husband to spend time together dining, but it really was taking its toll on her body. Sam's eating patterns were aligned with the children for the first part of the day, then she switched to her husband's schedule for the latter part. He would often have a large nutritious meal for lunch, but she would grab a quick Vegemite sandwich. Sam's food diary showed she was essentially grazing from the time she started preparing the children's dinner and would often end up eating a serving of theirs as well as hers later on.

I decided to take Sam to a resistance-training group exercise class as part of her exercise program. It happened to be at 7.30 p.m., so I asked her to eat a decent meal with the children before the class. When we met before class, she said she felt fantastic, had heaps of energy and realised it was her hunger making her so irritable every night. She performed brilliantly in the class (her first ever) and was so energised and inspired she stayed after class for an extra 20 minutes on the treadmill.

Sam emailed me later that night to say she had, upon returning home, immediately instructed her husband she would no longer be eating with him during the week. He may not have appreciated me at the time, but with a happier, healthier wife he can only win.

We also decided Sam could get away with cooking only three dinners a week. She'd cook a double quantity on Mondays and freeze half. On Tuesdays she would eat the frozen meal from the previous Monday (to avoid having the same meal two nights running). She would cook fresh meals on Wednesdays and Thursdays, enjoy takeaway on Fridays and her husband would cook both weekend nights. Easy!

PART III
Move it and lose it

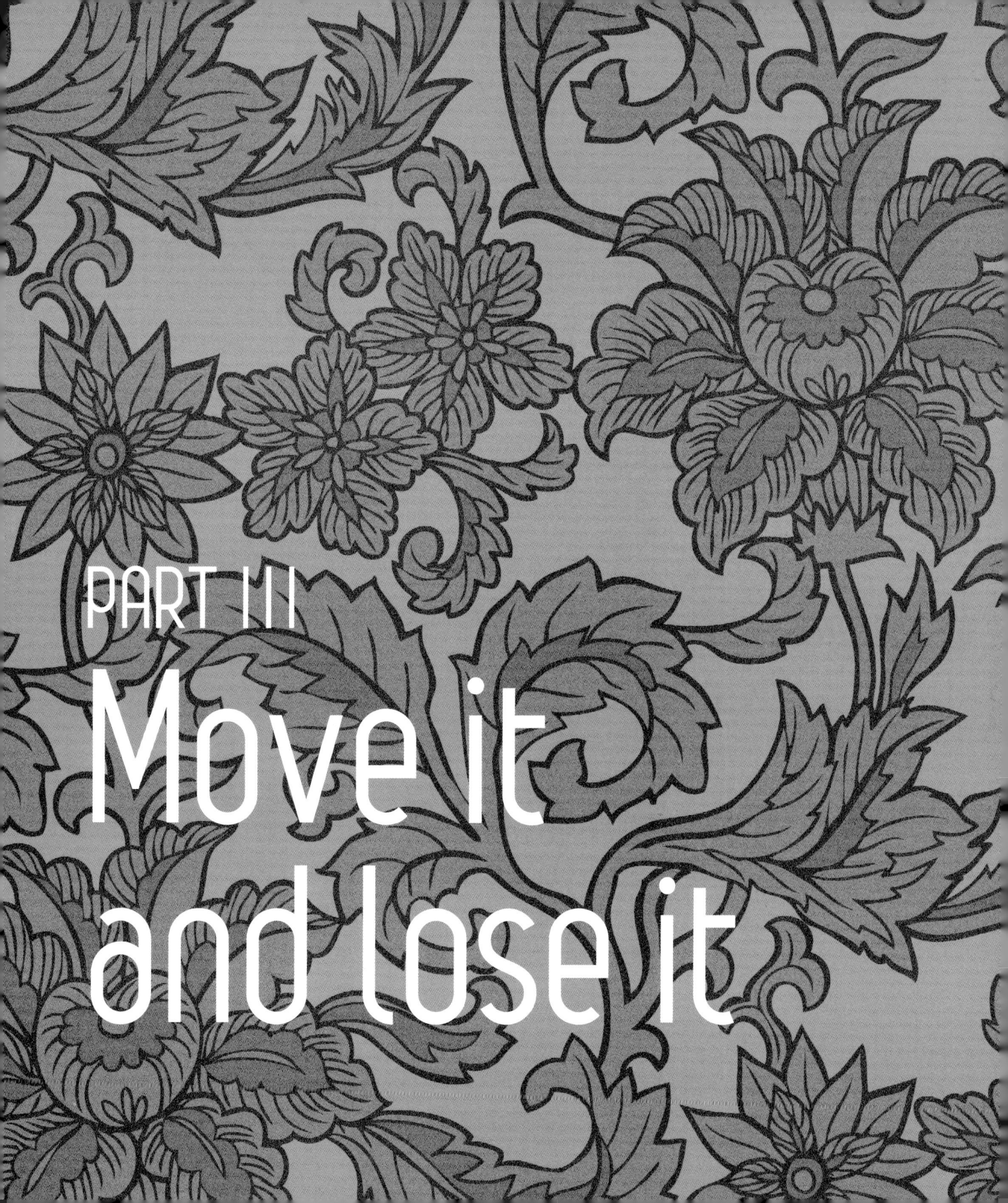

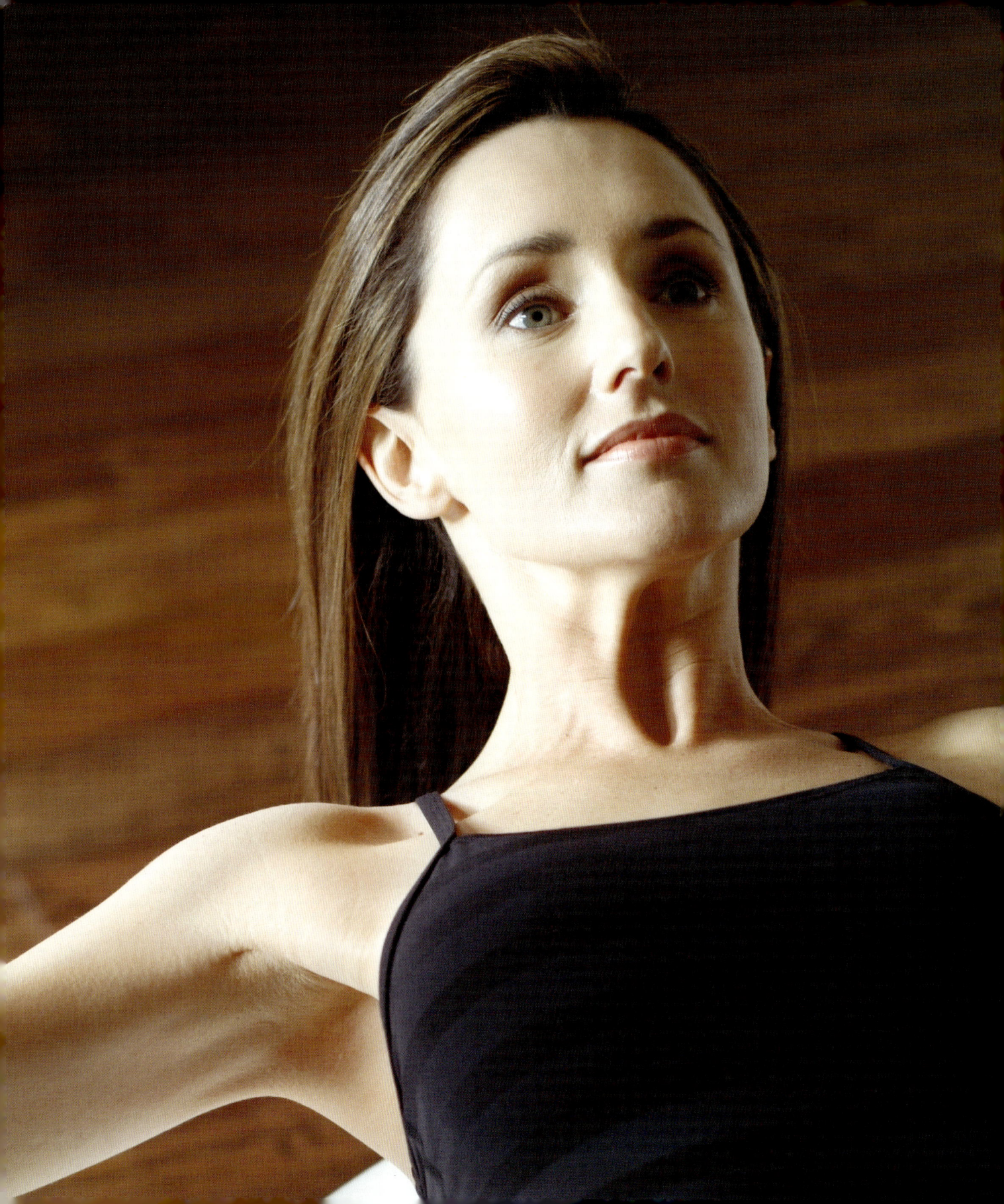

Facts about fitness

WHY EXERCISE?

Today . . .
- To feel great.
- To have energy to do what you need to do and what you want to do.
- To elevate your mood—endorphins are a great addiction!
- To relax and sleep well.
- To look great—your body *can* be better than you ever thought, even after babies.
- To have confidence in your body—both in and out of clothes!

Tomorrow . . .
- To live longer, with a better quality of life.
- To prevent or manage many common diseases including diabetes, coronary artery disease, osteoporosis.
- To stay strong, in mind and body.

If all this came in a pill, it would be a best-seller!

WHAT IS FITNESS?

Fitness can be defined in several ways. Most often it refers to how well your body performs in tests of speed, strength, suppleness, stamina and body composition. General fitness training concentrates on two main areas: cardiovascular fitness (stamina) and muscle strength.

Ready?

What's so great about exercise?

The different types of fitness—and how to get them

How often, hard and long should I exercise?

What is the best sort of exercise?

Fat-burning myths and facts

Introducing some basic fitness equipment

Setting goals to change your body for good

Cardiovascular fitness

Stamina is 'cardiovascular' or 'aerobic' fitness. Cardiovascular fitness literally means fitness of the heart and blood vessels. It refers to how efficiently your heart pumps blood around the body to deliver oxygen needed for energy production in the tissues. As you start to move, your heart beats faster in response to the increased demand for oxygen from your muscles. As you get fitter, your heart gets stronger and more efficient at pumping. Your blood vessels also get more effective at carrying and delivering blood, and your heart does not have to beat as fast to do the work. So a fitter person has a lower heart rate for any given activity, even rest; a lower resting heart rate is an indication of fitness.

Remember our twins from chapter 4—fit Sally and unfit Jane. Sally's heart rate while she's resting is 60 beats per minute. With every beat her left ventricle (a chamber in the heart) ejects a strong surge of richly oxygenated blood, which is carried through a dense capillary network to all her tissues. Jane's heart, on the other hand, ticks away at 78 beats per minute at rest. It has to work much harder to push her blood around as her whole cardiovascular system is less efficient.

Getting fit is what happens when you *repeatedly* stimulate your body (through exercise) to use fuel to provide energy for movement which raises your heart rate for a sustained period. Over time this results in a training effect—you get fitter. All systems for energy production and recruitment become more efficient and your body responds by building more tissue for storing fuel for exercise (muscle) and less tissue for storing fat.

When people lose a significant amount of weight and become fitter through exercise they feel great. It's not all about looks: when you're fit, and you carry more muscle than fat, you *feel* energetic. You surge through the day with vigour—a definite benefit for busy mums. Without fitness, you can feel overtired and overworked all the time—which in reality you probably are! But as the human body is an incredibly adaptable machine, by getting fitter you'll cope better with those sleepless nights and days constantly on the go. The fitter you get, the easier it is to get off the couch, because you're not so lethargic. You get used to moving, to exercising, to using your body, and your body adapts. Similarly, your body also quickly adapts to not moving and to neglect.

I've been on both sides: I've been very fit and very unfit. The unfit phases were my pregnancies, when I was very sick and immobile for so long. Initially I lost a lot of weight very quickly, but it was all muscle. I could hardly walk and had no energy at all. I gradually regained fitness after the births and the feeling was liberating, like I had awoken from a long, sluggish dream.

Being fit is also the best beauty treatment you can get! Your improved capillary network more efficiently supplies every inch of skin with hydration, vitamins, minerals and proteins. This works infinitely better than anything you can slap on the outside. Exercise really does keep you looking young. Take dance teachers for example. I've met many veteran dance instructors and you couldn't guess their age within 10 years in some cases. Well after 50, their skin is tight, their eyes are bright, they're full of energy and they have lean, supple limbs. This is a group for whom regular movement is a way of life, and they demonstrate the benefits of using the human body in accordance with how it was clearly designed.

Muscle strength and resistance training

Muscle strength can be improved by resistance training or strength training, which are interchangeable terms, as it involves training against resistance to gain strength.

In chapter 4 I mentioned that resistance training is the fit and fabulous mum's secret to a great body. Well, here it is: all women should use their muscles. Use it or lose it! After your body reaches full adult maturity in the early to mid-twenties, it's all downhill from there unless you actively use, maintain and improve what you have. This is particularly true for bones and muscles. We can slow or prevent bone-density loss (osteoporosis) with resistance training. Research shows that, unless we actively do something about it, we lose lean muscle tissue every year after the mid-twenties, but usually still gain weight. This means we put on fat. And the news gets worse after menopause: women store fat around the middle (like men), which significantly increases our risk of cardiovascular disease.

Many women worry about 'getting bigger' or looking too muscled if they do resistance training. However, the physique of an Olympic shot-putter or a professional female body-builder is incredibly hard to achieve for the average woman. A genetic predisposition, hormones (and possibly steroid supplements) and many, many hours of daily strenuous weight training can produce larger, muscled physiques in women. But it is very difficult. It's hard enough for some men to get the muscled physiques they want. Most women tell me when I prescribe exercise that they prefer the distinctly feminine but fit forms of a volleyball player or a ballroom dancer. These bodies are honed using a combination of cardiovascular exercise and high-repetition resistance training using lower weights, plus stretching and great nutrition, of course! I often get requests to help 'tone up'. This is a vague term, but refers to the look given by increased muscle definition, strength and shape—all achieved with weight training and losing fat.

Most women shun the idea of hitting the weights room at a gym with all the sweaty, grunting men, but this is not the only way to train with resistance. Chances are that you've done some type of resistance training before without even realising it. For example, swimming is resistance training. Your limbs are performing many repetitions of pulling and pushing to propel you against the resistance of the water, which builds strength and is also a great cardio workout. Cycling is good resistance work for the legs, particularly up hills or cross-country on a mountain bike. Gymnastics and dance have many moves that build strength using body weight as resistance, such as jumps, lunges, lifts, push-ups, handstands and other balance work.

The type of cardiovascular exercise you do may also provide resistance work to maintain muscle mass. But specific strength training will help you reach particular goals. A new mother has many muscles to rehabilitate and usually wants to alter her body composition—that is, lose the baby fat, which takes lean body mass (muscle) to accomplish. This means doing a series of exercises that overload the muscles and stimulate them to grow stronger. You need to pull, push, press or lift something against a force, which may be gravity or machinery. You can use your own body weight, dumbbells or free weights, resistance-training machines, exercise bands or tubes. The various options for exercise equipment are explained later in this chapter.

One thing I need to make absolutely clear is that exercises which work the muscles slowly, which are designed to increase strength and do not raise the heart rate significantly do not 'burn fat' in a specific area. There is a lot of misinformation surrounding this issue. People often try to decrease a particular area with an exercise like crunches for the abdominals or leg lifts for the thighs. This idea is called 'spot reduction' and it is a myth. The body does not work in this way.

The body stores and uses stored fat according to a genetic map and you cannot direct it otherwise. Abdominal exercises do not reduce the amount of fat on your stomach area. They will make the muscles *underneath* the fat layer strong and shapely, but no number of repetitions or 'ab training' equipment will give you a 'six-pack' or 'washboard' stomach. You have to reduce total body fat to decrease this or any other area. In fact many people have a six-pack—they just can't see it for the fat blanket on top! So there's no point doing thousands of leg lifts or thigh squeezes each day. To get the shape you want in particular areas like the legs or abdominals, you can do exercises to effectively overload the muscles in the area to get them strong and shapely, but you have to combine it with cardiovascular exercise to use the stored fat sitting on top of the muscles. And of course you have to make sure you create an energy deficit to use the stored fat.

During resistance training you use energy to perform the exercises, and there are ways to increase your heart rate and enhance the total energy used in your training sessions. By doing exercises that require large muscle groups (compound exercises) or alternating between upper and lower body exercises (called 'peripheral heart action' training) you can increase your heart rate. Also, alternating exercises instead of resting in between sets of the same exercise keeps you moving, keeps the blood pumping and saves you time. The chapters that follow show you how to exercise efficiently, giving optimal results for a minimal time commitment.

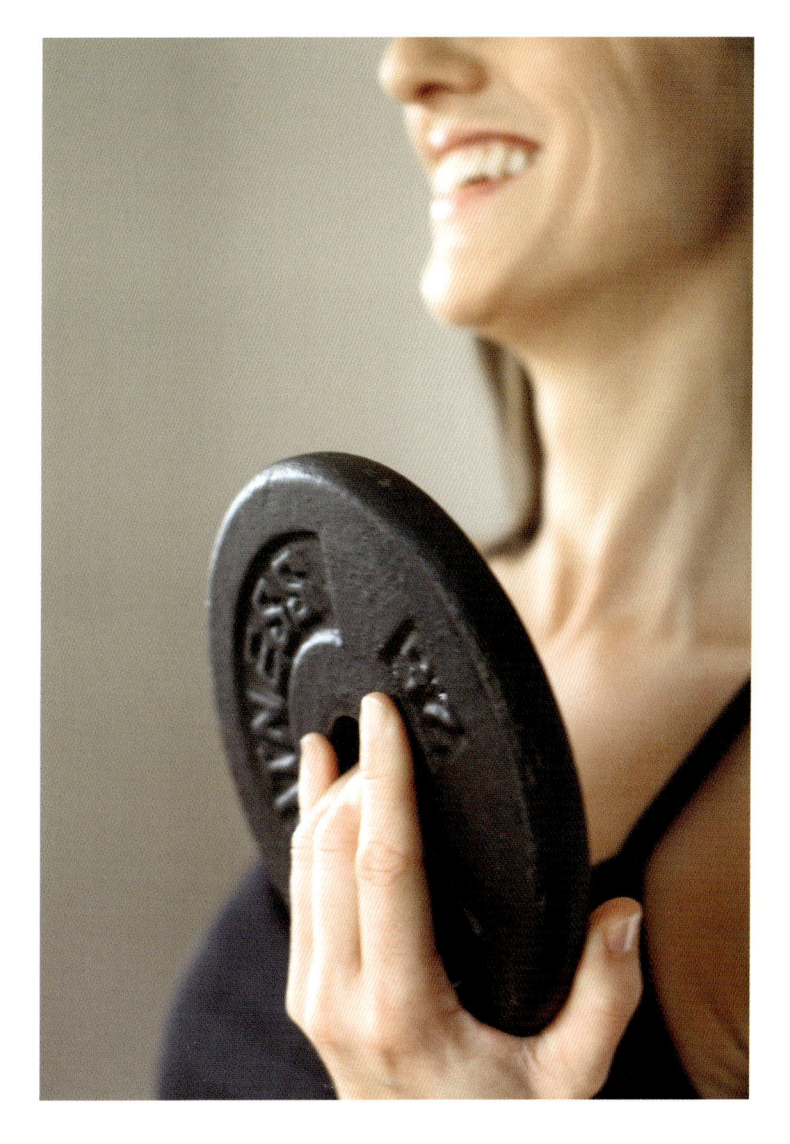

THE F.I.T.T. FORMULA

When prescribing cardiovascular exercise, the F.I.T.T. formula can be used to improve your heart health, use up body fat and get fit. It stands for frequency, intensity, time and type.

Frequency: how often you exercise, such as three times per week.
Intensity: how hard you work, from barely breaking a sweat to puffing and panting.
Time: how long the exercise session lasts.
Type: what sort of exercise you are doing, such as walking or swimming.

The National Heart Foundation recommends 30 minutes of moderate-intensity exercise on most, if not all, days. They advise brisk walking is ideal and you can accumulate 10 minutes at a time if it's more convenient (see www.heartfoundation.com.au). This is a very simple, effective but general fitness prescription.

The following sections explain how we can apply the F.I.T.T. formula to fit the lifestyle and goals of a new mum.

Frequency

Mothers of little ones feel they rarely get the chance to do anything not classified as immediately vital, such as exercise. This comes back to time management and planning. Once you get your schedule sorted out, try to fit in 30 minutes of exercise each day, *on average*. This may seem like a lot of 'spare' time to find, but note the term on average. If you get only 10 minutes one day, do extra the next day. You can do three 10-minute or two 15-minute sessions if you like. Thirty minutes a day adds up to only three and a half hours a week. So, if you walk three times a week for around an hour at a decent intensity, that would also be fine. Remember, the more you do, the faster you'll see results.

Daily exercise is great if you can get it, but with my two young ones and busy work schedule, I don't even do it every day. I prefer to block out a decent session several times a week, with alternatives for contingencies, but others prefer to break it down into smaller pieces.

The exercise chapters will give you a plan for what to do (including cardiovascular, strength and flexibility exercises) and how much to do; this is Plan A. But whatever you end up doing, put it in your schedule. Remember, Plan B is always better than nothing.

Intensity

For exercise to be effective, you have to work hard enough to produce the desired results. Miranda lives near the beach and tells me she swims and walks most days, eats well, but is not getting fitter and is actually putting on weight. On spending some time with Miranda and observing her 'workouts' I discover she is doing what she claims, but she's simply not working hard enough. Her walk is a short, comfortable stroll and the swimming is a leisurely paddle taking in the scenery. These leisurely activities are great for her, but she is staying in her comfort zone and will not get fitter without challenging her body. She needs to significantly raise her heart rate over a sustained period of time during her exercise sessions. This will get her fitter and increase her chance of losing weight.

When you start to exercise, the working muscles require more oxygen, which is delivered from the lungs through the bloodstream. So, the heart beats faster to pump the blood around more rapidly to keep up with the oxygen demand. The harder you work, the faster your breathing and heart rate. Heart rate is therefore an accurate way to measure exercise intensity.

The easiest way to measure your heart rate is to take your radial pulse by placing your index and middle fingers just below the inside of the wrist, below the thumb. You can also feel your pulse in the neck to one side of the windpipe. Using a watch with a second hand, count how many beats there are in one minute, or count for 15 seconds and multiply by four. At rest, counting for a minute is most accurate, as any error in counting for 15 seconds is also multiplied by four. However, if you're exercising, you usually have to stop or slow down to feel your pulse and over a minute your heart rate slows down too, so it won't be indicative of your exercise intensity. Stopping exercise for 15 seconds for a heart rate check is accurate enough.

TARGET HEART RATE

Your 'target heart rate' is what you aim to get your heart rate up to while exercising, for the most benefit. It is usually a percentage range of your assumed maximum heart rate and depends on your age and fitness level.

Recommendations on intensity vary, but generally, working in the range of 65–85 per cent of maximum heart rate is a good training zone. Use 65–75 per cent if you're starting out, and 75–85 per cent if you've been exercising and are fairly fit.

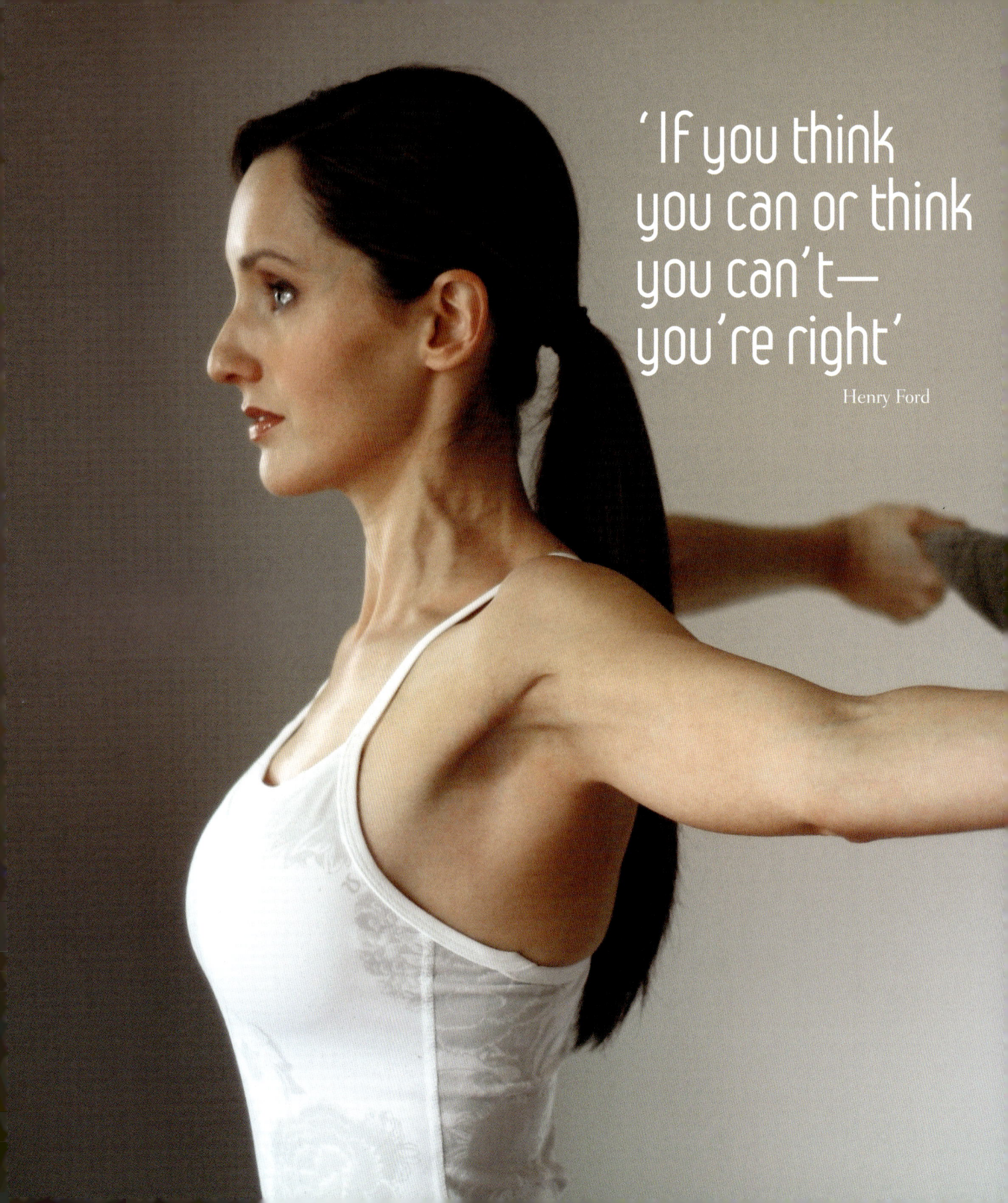

'If you think you can or think you can't— you're right'

Henry Ford

If you are sedentary, very unfit or overweight, an intensity of 60 per cent is enough until you build up your cardiovascular system. And you must get clearance from your doctor before starting this or any exercise recommendation, particularly if you have any complications such as diabetes, obesity, hypertension and coronary artery disease, or if you smoke. These types of conditions may require modifications to exercise intensities to ensure your safety.

A target heart rate for exercise is easy to calculate using the following formula:

[220 minus age] x 0.65 = target heart rate at 65% of maximum heart rate
Example for a 35-year-old:
[220 – 35] x 0.65 = [185] x 0.65 = 120.25 beats per minute
[220 – 35] x 0.75 = [185] x 0.75 = 138.75 beats per minute

So the target heart rate range at 65–75 per cent for a 35-year-old is 120–138 beats per minute. The number 220 is the maximum assumed heart rate at birth. As you get older and your heart gets bigger and stronger it beats more slowly, which is why you subtract your age from 220 for your maximum.

This formula, however, doesn't account for individual fitness level. If you are of average fitness for your age, then this formula will be close enough. But if you are very fit, your heart will be efficient, works like a younger heart and is capable of a higher maximum rate. Also, if you are very unfit, your heat beats faster for less work, as it is a weaker muscle and has a lower maximum rate.

As few of us are truly 'average', we can make this formula more specific to you with a simple modification called the Karvonen formula. Measure your resting heart rate as soon as you wake up in the morning, while still lying down. Put a watch and a reminder note beside your bed, as it can take a few days to remember! Recall that the lower your resting heart rate, the fitter you are, so measuring it periodically is a good way to monitor progress.

The Karvonen formula:

{[220 minus age] minus resting heart rate} x 0.65 + resting heart rate = target heart rate at 65% of maximum

Example for a 35-year-old with a resting heart rate of 68 beats per minute:
{[220 − 35] − 68} x 0.65 + 68 = 144.05
{[220 − 35] − 68} x 0.75 + 68 = 155.75

The target heart rate range at 65–75 per cent intensity is 145–155 beats per minute.

As you can see, accounting for individual fitness levels can make a big difference in the heart rate to aim for during exercise. So, to be as accurate and efficient as possible in your exercise, do the quick calculations, rather than using the guide for 'average' people.

PERCEIVING EXERTION

There are also simple subjective methods to estimate exercise intensity. The Rate of Perceived Exertion is a scale from 6 to 20 describing how intense exercise feels, from resting to feeling like your heart's about to explode (see Table 7.1).

A good working zone is 12–16, which roughly corresponds to about 120–160 beats per minute or 60–80 per cent of maximum heart rate. If you like this quick and easy method, you can practise to become more accurate with your 'guessing'. After picking a number, add a zero to it and then take your heart rate as well. See how close the numbers are. If you said 13 but your heart rate was only 110, you think you're working harder than you are! You'll then know what an 11 feels like, and you'll have to work harder to get to 13. This method seems a bit vague but can be surprisingly accurate.

You can also try a scale of 1–10 if you don't like the 6–20 range. This relates directly to a percentage, which you can calculate using the Karvonen formula. So, you can aim to work as hard as a 7 or 8 out of 10 and this should correspond to 70–80 per cent of maximum heart rate. And again, you can check the accuracy of your perception by taking your heart rate.

Doing the calculations and experiencing exercising at the right intensity to get results is useful primarily as a learning tool. Once you know what it *should* feel like, you don't need to monitor heart rate

TABLE 7.1

RATE OF PERCEIVED EXERTION

6	resting
7–8	very, very light exertion
9–10	very light exertion
11–12	fairly light exertion
13–14	somewhat hard exertion
15–16	hard exertion
17–18	very hard exertion
19–20	very, very hard exertion

constantly. Checking it every six weeks or so is sufficient to track the effects of exercise.

The easiest way to tell if you're exercising hard enough is the 'talk test'. If you can sing while exercising, the intensity is light. If you can have a conversation, the intensity is moderate. If you're too out of breath to talk at all, it is vigorous. Based on this, most people are comfortable with moderate intensity, but if you want to challenge yourself, throw in some short intervals of vigorous intensity now and then.

When considering exercise intensity, take into account that you need to work hard enough to get results, but not so hard that you don't enjoy it. Particularly when starting exercise, it's more important to create the habit and stick to the program than to get your heart rate to the target intensity each time.

MYTHS ABOUT INTENSITY AND FAT-BURNING

These are two of the biggest exercise myths you've probably heard:

- You have to exercise at a lower intensity to burn more fat. False. Lower intensities use a higher percentage of fuel from fat, but lower total kilojoules and lower total fat than more intense activities.
- You don't start burning fat until 20 minutes into an exercise session. False. We always use a mix of fat and carbohydrate fuel—the mix changes depending on the intensity. More total time spent exercising uses more total kilojoules. It does not matter whether it's one 30-minute session or three 10-minute sessions.

Consider the following facts about how our bodies use fuel during exercise.

- At all times, we use a combination of carbohydrates and fats as fuel for exercise and other activities. These fuels need oxygen to 'burn', to produce energy.
- To burn or use fat energy requires more oxygen than carbohydrate, and is considered 'slow burning'. As exercise intensity increases, your heart rate and breathing get faster to keep up with the oxygen demand, but it gets harder to deliver oxygen quickly enough to the working muscles.
- Carbohydrates can be used with lesser amounts of oxygen available and are a 'fast-burning' fuel, good for higher energy demands at higher intensities.

When you exercise at lower intensities or rest, you use a larger *proportion* of fat as fuel, and as intensity increases, you use a larger *proportion* of carbohydrate as fuel. But since you use *greater total energy* in a higher-intensity workout, you most probably burn more *total fat* and definitely use more kilojoules, increasing the chance of tipping the energy equation to favour weight loss.

Compare the three workouts below.

Workout 1: Walking for one hour, a female of 67 kg burns 1000 kJ, of which 60% is fat and 40% is carbohydrate.
Total fat kJ used = 60% x 1000 kJ = 600 kJ
Total carbohydrate kJ used = 40% x 1000 kJ = 400 kJ

Workout 2: Running for one hour, the same 67 kg female burns 2000 kJ, of which 40% is fat and 60% is carbohydrate.
Total fat kJ used = 40% x 2000 kJ = 800 kJ
Total carbohydrate kJ used = 60% x 2000 kJ = 1200 kJ

No workout: Resting with a book for an hour, the same 67 kg female burns 300 kJ, of which 80% is fat and 20% is carbohydrate.
Total fat kJ used = 80% x 300kJ = 240kJ
Total carbohydrate kJ used = 20% x 300kJ = 60kJ

So, along with the benefits of challenging the cardiovascular system and getting fitter, you use more kilojoules and are more likely to burn stored body fat (and create an energy deficit) at higher exercise intensities.

However, it's often more appropriate, safer or more comfortable to exercise at lower intensities if you are a beginner, overweight or obese, or suffer from hypertension or coronary artery disease, for example. The best strategy is to increase your exercise *time* to use more total energy. If you plan a 15-minute jog, but don't feel like running, walk for 30 minutes instead.

Aerobics classes and videos often perpetuate these myths with 'fat-burner' classes, which are usually low-intensity and low-impact beginner-level classes. They are a great place to start exercising, but you would burn more total fat in a harder workout, as seen in the example workouts.

The best fat-burning activity of all is the one you'll do the most often, as the key to weight loss is sustained energy deficit through using up more energy than you eat.

INTERVAL TRAINING

Interval training is a great way to increase fitness, work up to higher intensities and use more kilojoules. All you have to do is work harder for short bursts during your exercise session. Add a few hills to your walking route, or scatter some one-minute sprints throughout a jog. On a stationary bike, you can increase the resistance for 'hills'. Whatever you're doing, start with one short interval of harder work. Then go back to your normal pace. When you feel you have recovered, go hard again. Over the weeks, add more frequent and longer intervals to your workout. It will get easier, which means you are getting fitter, and you'll see results.

Raising the intensity of exercise not only burns more kilojoules for the energy needed at the time, but it raises your metabolic rate and your temperature, which must be regulated. This uses extra energy after exercise for as long as it takes your body to return to resting conditions. This is called 'post-exercise energy consumption' and can be enhanced by increasing the intensity or duration of your workout.

INTENSITY CONSIDERATIONS FOR BREASTFEEDING

If you're breastfeeding you need to be aware of a by-product of high-intensity exercise called lactic acid. During heavy weight training or high-intensity cardiovascular work such as cycling uphill, your muscles may need to burn carbohydrate energy even if sufficient oxygen isn't delivered quickly enough. This process generates lactic acid and gives a 'burning' feeling in the muscles.

Lactic acid circulates through the bloodstream and is filtered out by the kidneys, and it does pass into breast milk. It does not hurt the baby, but she may fuss or even refuse a feed if the milk is too acidic. Lactic acid usually dissipates from the body in about two hours, and drinking plenty of water helps dilute it.

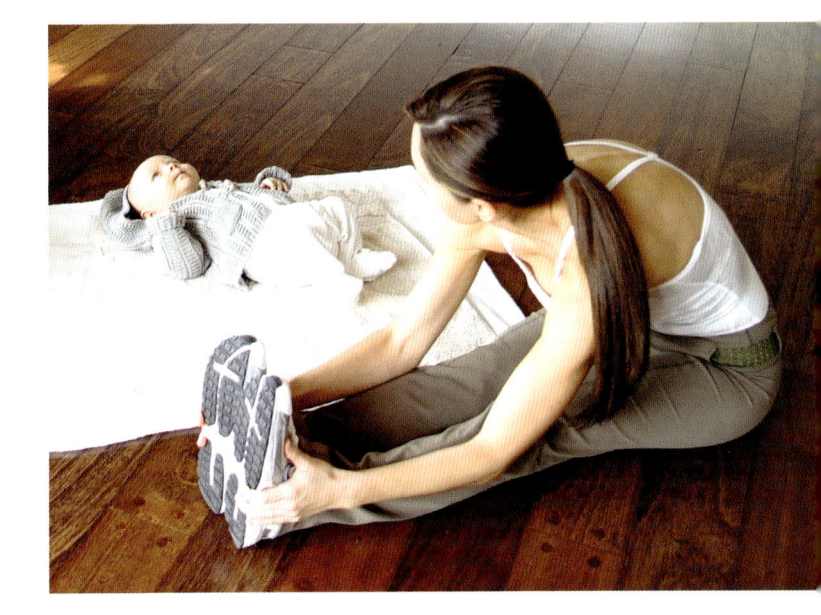

If you want strenuous workouts and baby is not happy with your post-exercise milk, try to time your workout after a feed. Then use expressed milk or formula for the next feed, and discard milk produced directly after exercise. I didn't encounter this problem (I mustn't have exercised hard enough!), but feeding mothers who are competitive athletes may consider this. And keep in mind that too much exercise or losing weight too quickly could diminish your milk supply, so listen to your body and your baby and don't go overboard.

Time

With young children around you can get a lot of incidental exercise—unplanned physical activity that just happens during the course of the day as you're going about your business. But if your aim is to get fitter and move stored body fat, you'll have to spend some time with your heart up in that target training zone. As already mentioned, the general recommendation is for 30 minutes of moderate exercise every day. If you can manage more, excellent. This may include time spent walking to work, local shops or school, but aim for moderate intensity, not an easy stroll.

And remember, you can accumulate 30 minutes in blocks of 10 or 15 minutes. However, there are some benefits to doing 30 minutes or more in one hit. When aiming for a moderate intensity, it can take a couple of minutes to get into it, warm up and set a good pace, then 10 minutes is over before you know it. And if you exercise hard enough to get a bit of a 'glow' or even a decent sweat, it's more convenient to do it once a day when you can change or shower afterwards. Also, several smaller bursts of exercise are easily overlooked if they don't have a particular time slot allocated.

If you don't get 30 minutes every day, keep active anyway: walk as much as you can, run around after the children at the park, put music on and dance at home (this always amuses toddlers), and make up for it with longer sessions when you can.

The main consideration is fitting it into your schedule, making a realistic plan for when and how long you can exercise, and not making excuses when the time comes around!

Type of exercise

The best form of exercise is the one you'll do, and do most often! There is no one best exercise for everyone and it depends on your goals. No two exercise plans are identical, even if the goals are the same, because no two people are the same. There are so many contributing and limiting factors, such as age, injuries, general health, exercise history, personal preferences, abilities and schedule.

In the exercise chapters I prescribe a program combining cardiovascular and resistance exercise tailored to a specific group with specific needs: rehabilitation, fitness and change in body composition after having babies.

Within this program you will still need to determine what type of cardiovascular exercise suits you best, and you might modify some resistance exercises. The various types of exercise have different benefits and risks which need to be weighed. The following summaries outline the major considerations for different types of exercise to help you consider which ones to try. Remember, the human body was designed and built for movement, and regular exercise is critical to lifelong health and getting in shape after babies. So, accept that you need to move, then consider not if, but how, you'll do it . . .

WEIGHT-SUPPORTED AND WEIGHT-BEARING EXERCISE

Most forms of cardiovascular exercise can be grouped into two main categories:

- **Weight-supported:** your weight is carried for you and you repetitively push against a source of resistance.
- **Weight-bearing:** you support and carry your own body weight.

As well as the benefits of cardiovascular exercise, they both provide a degree of resistance training, with benefits for bones and muscles. All forms of cardiovascular exercise involve using muscles to move and hence raising your heart rate as the demand for oxygen in the working muscles increases.

Some forms of cardiovascular exercise provide light resistance training for certain muscle groups. An example of this is cycling. It is weight-supported (the bike carries your body weight), but you push against the resistance of the tyres on the ground. This gets harder off-road or up hills as these options provide more resistance. A trained cyclist will have relatively smaller upper body muscles, yet strong, developed leg muscles.

Swimming is another form of weight-supported exercise, as the water provides buoyancy, and you push your way through it. Water resistance is hard to work against, and the faster you move limbs through the water, the harder it gets. So swimming raises the heart rate which increases cardiovascular fitness, and also provides strength gains in specific muscle groups used—arms, shoulders, legs, torso, depending on the stroke.

Exercise equipment where you sit down—such as rowing machines, stationary bikes and recumbent cycles (with a back rest, and legs out in front)—are all weight-supported, and you can alter the resistance on the machine to determine how hard you work.

Walking, jogging, dancing and gymnastics are forms of weight-bearing exercise, because you carry the weight of your body as you move. When walking, for example, you can increase the intensity by going faster, going up hills, carrying baby in a pouch or pushing a pram.

Weight-bearing exercises provide benefits for bone and muscle strength. Research has shown that bone strength is increased or maintained by repetitively putting force on them (impact). Gymnasts, for example, show increased bone density in their forearms and forelegs due to habitual jumping, landing, tumbling and handsprings. What that means for non-athletes is that we can maintain our bones and muscles effectively by carrying our own weight around as we walk, jog, jump rope or play tennis.

WHAT IS THE IMPACT OF WEIGHT-BEARING EXERCISE?

You may have heard the terms 'low impact' or 'high impact' in reference to exercise, particularly if you got into the early-90s aerobics craze. Impact is the force of hitting something, and in exercise it is usually your foot hitting the ground. But the force does not stop at the point of impact (your foot); it also affects the rest of your body. Impact from jumping is sustained through the foot, the ankle, knee and hip joints, through the spine, right up to where the neck supports the head—it's all connected. So you need to consider the extra stress placed on joints, bones and cartilage during repetitive, high-impact activity.

Although some weight-bearing exercise helps bones become and stay strong, too much impact can compromise the weak points—the joints. The function of joints is to allow movement. Joint stability is provided by the ligaments which cross over the joint, attaching bones together. Tendons, which attach muscles to bones, also provide support. If the aim of exercise is to increase mobility and fitness, you don't want to risk permanent injury, immobility or disability. It's about moderation, monitoring, appropriate choices and cross training, the latter of which is addressed shortly.

High-impact activities include jogging, running, gymnastics, tennis, basketball and jumping rope. What these have in common is flight: both feet leave the ground at some point, allowing your entire body weight to land on one or both feet, repetitively. This is magnified by the force of gravity, so the higher you jump, the harder you land, and the greater the impact.

Examples of low-impact activities are walking, cycling, stepping, skating, swimming and rowing. The common element is that there is one foot on the ground at all times, or the body weight is supported. Activities like dancing and aerobics, where the moves are varied, are usually a combination of high and low impact, depending how hard you work.

Impact is also influenced by the surface on which you are exercising. Fitness facilities install sprung wooden floors in group exercise rooms; these are also used for dance and gymnastics. There is considerably less impact in landing on this type of flooring compared to a concrete slab. Soccer played on a grassy field has less impact than on any hard floor, but speed, momentum and collisions provide their own risks.

High-impact activities tend to be more intense and build a greater cardiovascular fitness than low-impact types, but the risks of acute or overuse injuries are greater, such as the ankle and knee injuries common in basketball. While one of the toughest things you can do to your body is to run solely on hard surfaces such as concrete or bitumen, many people run regularly on roads for years with no adverse effects.

When considering high-impact activities, you need to weigh long-term benefits against risks. Pick one you enjoy, which gives a good workout, and take steps to minimise injury—for example, good footwear, appropriate for the sport or activity, will support and protect your feet and absorb impact. Also, assess your options. A treadmill—especially one with a sprung deck—is a safe, even surface and lower impact compared to a road or path. You can listen to music and just go hard, without worrying about dodging potholes, bikes or cars. Walking or jogging cross-country or off-road—on sand, playing fields, parks or bush tracks—is a great workout because of the variations in slope and surface, but you must pay attention to your footing.

Remember too that if you are pregnant or have recently had a baby, your risks of impact-related injuries are greater. During pregnancy, your balance is compromised, some important core support muscles are impaired and a hormone (relaxin) contributes to joint instability. Add this to the stress of carrying extra body and baby weight and it's wise to keep impact minimal and movements controlled.

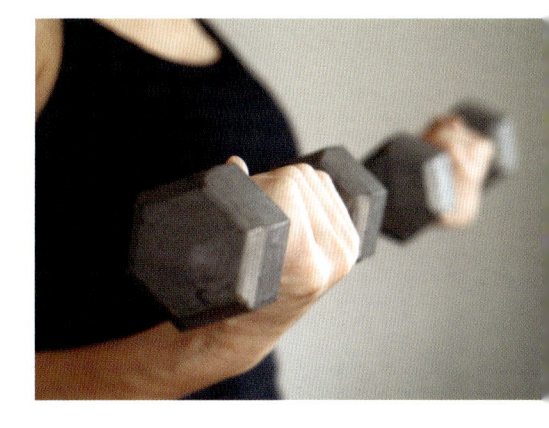

A low-impact workout does not necessarily mean low intensity. There are many ways to increase your heart rate without jarring your joints. For example, walk faster, like a race-walker—pump your arms, take powerful steps and go up hills. For a real challenge, add the weight of pushing a pram—I push a twin pram and with my two, their drinks and toys, the whole package now outweighs me!—but keep off roads.

I don't recommend walking with hand or ankle weights. They are too light for decent strength training or to considerably increase the heart rate, yet are heavy enough to stress the joints when swinging vigorously from the end of limbs. Any movements with added weight must be done *under muscular control* for safety and effectiveness. Using weights with momentum is not recommended unless under the supervision of an exercise physiologist for specific sports-training purposes like a golf swing. Anyway, the extra weight from hand weights is so small that you easily use more energy by walking faster, further or up a hill.

Light hand weights are sometimes used in aerobics classes, and if movements are kept slow in speed and low in impact, then they can safely help raise heart rate for those who don't want to run and jump. But the emphasis is on *controlled* movement. It is practically impossible not to swing your arms if you're walking fast—and if you're swinging, you're using momentum, not muscle control. People do it assuming it 'tones' the arms, but only slow movements and heavier weights which challenge the muscles achieve this. I recommend a fast-paced walk up a hill instead, and then home for a couple of strength exercises with real resistance for real results.

If you want to carry something to increase your heart rate without going faster, carry a backpack or something designed to fit on the body for safer carrying as opposed to swinging from the end of a limb. You can walk with a baby pouch as long as it fits your body well and doesn't hurt your back. This is a form of progressive training; you become stronger and get a better workout as baby gets heavier.

If you do a dance class, a low-impact fitness class or DVD, use large and exaggerated moves and really get into it. Take big steps, lift your knees high and use your arms through their full range of movement above the head. This will get your heart rate higher. Also try to do it on flooring such as timber or carpet rather than tiles or concrete.

Water is the ultimate all-round, no-impact workout. Whether you're paddling along with a kickboard, doing an aqua-fitness class or speeding through laps in a beautiful butterfly stroke, you can't go wrong in the pool.

Many people assume water workouts are only for the elderly, the injured, the pregnant or the obese. Not true! If you have access to a pool you'll be surprised how hard you can work, how great you'll feel and how soon you'll want to do it again. Even 'non-swimmers' can get a great, safe workout in the pool.

Exercise equipment such as steppers, rowing machines, stationary bikes and elliptical trainers all give you a great workout with minimal impact on your body. In-line skating or rollerskating is also low impact (unless you're doing stunts or jumps).

Few of us are entirely free of physical limitation throughout our lives. Besides pregnancy, there are many reasons you may alter your exercise plan, such as injury, illness, surgery, or diseases like hypertension, diabetes, arthritis or cardiovascular disease. In many cases, however, you can still exercise and it is important to seek out options with your health care professional. Exercise can help manage the symptoms of many conditions, while inactivity can compound them.

Cross training

Constantly challenging your body stimulates it to become fitter. Cross training—regularly participating in more than one type of exercise—helps you achieve balanced fitness and minimises overuse or repetitive strain injuries. An example of cross training is combining cardiovascular exercise with resistance training and stretches in your weekly routine.

I constantly refer to the human body as being very adaptable. Increasing fitness is an example of this. If you exercise, your body adapts by becoming fitter and stronger to cope with the repeated exercise sessions. But your body gets used to exercise too, and you can reach a plateau where you may not be getting fitter or losing more weight. Getting your heart rate up using different muscle groups is the perfect way to reinvent a 'stale' exercise schedule and keep you interested. And if you challenge your body in a way to which it is not accustomed, this uses more energy than your usual exercise. If you usually just walk, add a swim or some weights once a week. Or if you use a rowing machine three times this week, next week jog with the pram twice and do yoga.

If you get stuck for ideas on keeping your exercise program 'fresh', don't forget to check out local community colleges and centres, schools and hospitals—they have some great, well-priced adult classes which run to school terms. You only have to commit for 8–10 weeks (unlike gym memberships), you can try a variety of new activities and often find like-minded friends in the process. Have you ever tried martial arts, belly dancing, fencing or hiking?

Initially, the best activity is the one you'll do, and keep doing, to form an exercise habit. Then once that's nailed, modify your plan to help you achieve more specific goals.

DON'T FORGET TO STRETCH!

This area of fitness is often overlooked. Tight muscles, even if strong, can limit range of motion and increase risk of injury and muscle imbalance. Try this simple flexibility test. Sit on the floor with your legs stretched out in front of you. If you can't reach your toes—you need work in this area!

Every time you move or hold a posture, your muscles contract (shorten and tighten) to move bones or stabilise them. This happens in any position other than lying down—while walking, feeding baby, sitting at a desk or exercising. Flexibility training, or stretching, keeps muscles working effectively through a full range of motion, relaxes them and improves your posture.

Pregnancy and caring for babies is physically demanding work which can give you tight, aching muscles. A sore, tight lower back with poor support (due to weak abdominal muscles), tight leg muscles from sitting a lot, and knots in your shoulders and neck from feeding, settling and carrying baby are all common complaints from new mums.

Stretching is quick and simple to slot in any time and can make a big difference to how your body feels and performs. Stretching in between strength exercises saves time and is also effective, as muscles stretch better when warm. Muscles are elastic: if you put a rubber band in the freezer you'll see it doesn't stretch much when cold, and usually breaks. So stretching after a walk or warm shower is both efficient and relaxing.

Yoga and Pilates are excellent, challenging activities for flexibility and strength. But if you want weight loss, you also need an activity that gets the heart rate up and uses lots of energy.

The exercise chapters in this book include stretches for the whole body. When stretching, follow the guidelines below.

Guidelines for stretching

- Ease into a stretch and hold it for 45–60 seconds. Do the same stretch three times with a short break in between; you'll get better.
- Hold the stretch where you feel resistance or tightness. Discomfort is okay, pain is not. If you are pregnant or within three months after giving birth, do not force stretches beyond your normal pre-pregnancy range. This can lead to loose joints, due to the hormone relaxin in the body.
- Exhale as you go into the stretch, continue to breathe and relax into the stretch and don't hold your breath.
- Never perform 'ballistic' or bouncing movements at the end of a stretch as this increases the risk of injury.
- Stretch all sides of the body; left, right, front and back. The aim is balance.
- Do a stretch or two whenever you can—stretch in the shower, when you go to bed, when you wake up, while watching TV and after feeding baby to loosen up. This stops you becoming a big bag of knots by the end of the week.

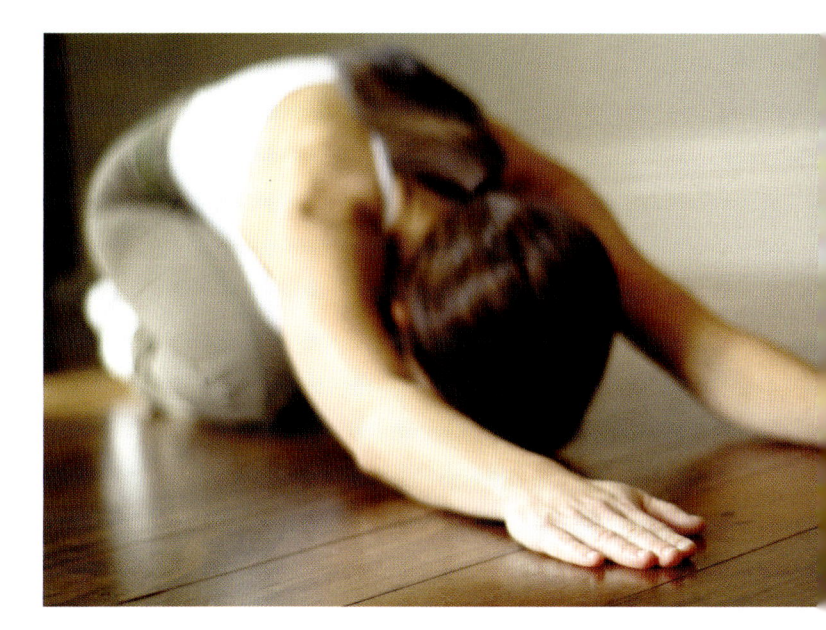

THE PROS AND CONS OF JOINING A GYM

Having worked for over 12 years in fitness centres on both sides of the Pacific, I know you can get great results *if you go regularly*. The facilities, instruction, range of exercise options and 'extras' like the cafe, spa or massage therapy can be motivating—if you have the time and budget!

Finding the time to go to a gym is a major issue. If you're at home all day with a baby, by the time your partner gets home you hardly feel like heading off to the gym, especially if it is more than 10 minutes drive from home. And babies are not great at fitting their feeding schedule around the class you want to do, either.

The biggest problem I have with commercial fitness centres is the membership fees. The longer your contract period, the cheaper it gets—but you're locked into paying for something which may not even fit your ever-changing lifestyle in three months, let alone three years! Many people wrongly assume that paying for a gym membership or fitness equipment will give them the motivation they require to keep going and achieve their fitness goals. This may last a month, if you're lucky!

Gyms are a good option for a busy mum if you find a facility with good child care and which offers a casual rate (pay-as-you-go) or a 10-visit pack, for example. You can still schedule three sessions a week and if you make it, great! But if you don't go for two weeks because someone's teething and someone else got a nasty cold and they all want mummy, you're not wasting money and feeling guilty about that *and* about not exercising. If your local fitness centre doesn't offer casual rates, keep asking until they do. Community facilities or local recreation centres are more likely to have casual rates. Even though the interior design may not be as appealing, they probably have all the equipment you need for a good workout. And the environment will be less intimidating than expensive fitness clubs full of gym junkies who dress up to be seen on the 'scene'.

An occasional consultation with an exercise physiologist to design an appropriate program to do at home is more cost-effective than a gym membership at this stage in your life, and is now subsidised by Medicare. Or you can simply follow the program described in this book and make the suggested changes as you get fitter.

HOME EQUIPMENT TO GET YOU MOVING

You can design a no-fail exercise program by being realistic about what you like to do, what you're willing to do and what you're able to manage. This section outlines some of the best exercise options for new mums.

The most important piece of workout equipment is the brain, not a collection of 'fitness' gadgets. I recommend creating the exercise habits first with the right information and tools to apply it. Then, as a reward, get yourself a useful piece of equipment or a 20-visit pass to a gym to boost your workouts. If you start by fostering success in smaller steps and create the habits first, you have a much greater chance of staying with exercise, whether at the gym or elsewhere.

When starting out, your body is the only piece of equipment you really need—you just need to know how to use it. Dancers, gymnasts and martial artists all train primarily using their own body weight, and they arguably have some of the most admired physiques for women and men.

However, a couple of simple key pieces of equipment can make achieving fitness goals easier and more enjoyable if you know what to get and how to use it.

A 'cardio' machine (equipment for cardiovascular training), such as a treadmill, rowing machine or stationary bike, has many advantages for a new mum. You can easily get 30 minutes of exercise in, at a decent intensity, when baby is sleeping. Or, provided baby is safely confined in a bouncer, rocker, pram, high chair or playpen, she may enjoy watching you exercise. Although walking outside is a great option, sometimes it's too hot, too cold, too wet, too dark or simply more trouble than it's worth to get you and baby out the door. Convenience helps dismiss excuses when you have limited exercise opportunities—and there is no more convenient place than home.

When my first baby was born, we lived in an area with no safe walking paths. So I got a treadmill on a rent-to-buy program that was particularly useful for the first six months after both my children were born. Renting was a great way to see if we'd use it, which both my husband and I did regularly enough to keep renting. After a year, we paid out the purchase price, as another six months' rental would have equalled it anyway. Ours is a middle-of-the-road treadmill—good enough to take a pounding from a decent-sized guy, but not commercial quality. It has a manual incline, variable speed, heart rate monitor (of questionable accuracy) and air-sprung deck. It folds easily and is light enough for me to move by myself. It fits all my essential criteria and six years later is still going strong. Not a bad investment in our health—and much cheaper than gym memberships for both of us.

Whether you like to jog, step or row, you don't have to pay retail for exercise equipment. The 'For Sale' section of the local paper, garage sales and online auctions are good sources for all types of exercise equipment. Ask your friends, colleagues and family, as you never know what people have lying around.

You don't need a whole room for a home gym, just an area to store a few things safely away from little fingers—under your bed, in a closet, behind the couch, somewhere with easy everyday access. Don't store exercise equipment in the garage—it's where unused household goods go to die. And don't buy fad pieces of equipment that look great on infomercials—you don't need anything but your body to train abdominals effectively, so forget this month's 'fab abs' contraption.

An exercise ball is the best thing for more challenging and varied abdominal work—it may look like a faddish gizmo, but it is actually a very good training tool. This big bouncy ball, originally used in rehabilitation, has become a mainstream fitness industry item. It's a ball, seat, bench and stretching rack all in one.

An exercise ball is great for 'core training', which means everything between your neck and your pelvis—which is what a new mother really needs. Exercises done on the ball are more challenging than on the ground as the ball is an unsteady base—the air in it displaces as you push against it, and this forces you to use more muscles to stabilise yourself. You can also use the ball with exercise bands or free weights. The range of exercises you can do is extensive and adaptable to any fitness level, and the ball itself is not expensive (I recently picked one up brand new at a recycled baby-goods store for $10!). I have included some ball work later in the exercise chapters.

Exercise tubes and bands are long pieces of rubber that come in different thicknesses and lengths for different amounts of resistance. Bands generally don't have handles, but tubes do. They are both easy to store and pack for travel. They are good for beginners or rehabilitation to work safely through a new exercise. However, they don't provide much resistance, the resistance is inconsistent and too hard to monitor, and it's too easy to cheat on the exercises. They're often used in group exercise situations as it's easier and safer to supervise 30 people using tubes rather than free weights.

Free weights (or dumbbells) are my number-one choice for resistance training—the guys have it right! They are portable and easily stored, can be adjustable, have a huge range of exercises for the whole body and use more muscles compared with weight-training machines as you have to stabilise the movement yourself. The main disadvantage is that many exercises require professional instruction to ensure safety and effectiveness and they can take a while to get used to. It is common for free-weight exercises to be done incorrectly. Weight machines restrict your range of motion to a specific exercise, which can make them safer, but the training options and results from free weights make it well worth learning correct training techniques.

For free weights to work, you need to lift them slowly against gravity. By changing body positions you use different muscle groups. The ball is handy for this, as is a chair or bench. An adjustable step bench is versatile, easily stored and can be used for lunging or stepping (cardio exercise) and to lie or sit on for weight training.

Although I've promoted the convenience of exercising at home, you should also get outdoors. That's right: fresh air, a change of scenery and some fast walking will do wonders for you and baby. You can feel very isolated, trapped or bored if you don't leave the house for days or weeks at a time. It's important to get out and interact with the world beyond your walls. By the time I had my second baby, my first was nearly two and we had moved to an area which is excellent for walking, so I got a great double pram and hit the pavement.

A great pram is absolutely the best piece of exercise equipment for a new mum! It gives you freedom and makes exercise easy and effective. It may seem odd, but I've had at least 12 prams and strollers, scouring online auctions, garage sales and second-hand baby-goods stores for my fleet. I borrowed from my friends and tried before I bought. I swapped, traded and upgraded. I have made money on some, particularly selling them online. I never had more wheels than I needed for the ages and stages of my children, but I quickly learned that the big, comfy prams great for newborn naps are not much good for walking on uneven footpaths, while the cross-country jogging pram was painful in the grocery store.

There are several good all-round prams on the market, which aren't too big for the shops but have good enough stability and appropriate wheels for fast walking as well. When my babies had enough head control, I graduated them to the small, light umbrella-fold stroller for quick outings such as shopping, and the fantastic bicycle-wheeled running pram for exercise. Now I'm instantly recognised around my neighbourhood with my bright purple twin running pram with huge wheels, and my shaggy little dog jogging alongside. With an aluminium frame it's light to steer, it's stable on all surfaces and holds something like 40 kg in each seat. I bought it second hand in mint condition in an online auction, where I paid about 20 per cent of the new price. It's kept me fit and the children happy as we head out most afternoons with their drinks and a snack for a look around the neighbourhood, which often includes a stop at the park. Even friends who thought I was obsessive have seen my point after borrowing my various prams. Anything which makes it easier to get out the door for a decent walk is worth the investment in your health . . . so when grandparents and friends ask what you'd like for the baby, set up a registry for the best-performing pram on the market!

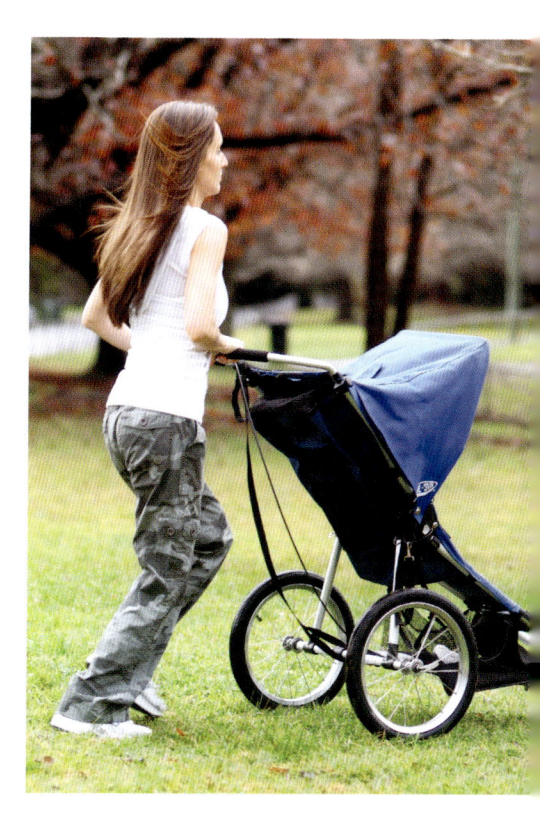

> ### The equipment wish list
>
> ❖ A pair of well-fitting shoes, suited to the activity you're doing.
> ❖ A great walking pram which fits as many children as you need to get out the door regularly.
> ❖ An exercise ball—check on the box that it's the right size for your height, and inflate at home with a foot pump.
> ❖ A small collection of free weights (dumbbells)—an adjustable set to share with your partner is best.
> ❖ Exercise videos for ideas and variety—yoga, Pilates, kickboxing, ballroom dancing.
> ❖ Cardio equipment such as a treadmill or rowing machine—on loan if possible, until you know you'll use it.

Once you're exercising regularly, put together a wish list of some useful pieces to boost your training. Some you may want before you start (like good walking shoes and a pram), but others you can save as rewards for your training efforts or for birthday presents. Better still, give them to your partner for his birthday. He won't suspect the weights are for you too, and he may shape up as well—another present for you!

SETTING FITNESS GOALS

The post-baby body can be a scary thing for the unsuspecting. During the pregnancy, you've had time to adjust to the expanding waistline. After baby's born, all of a sudden the tummy's empty, but it's still there and your breasts swell to the size of watermelons. Then over the next few months your body changes shape again. There's skin wrinkling and breasts shrinking, fat sticking where you'd rather it wouldn't, veins popping, hair falling out in clumps and some of your bones don't seem to be in the same place they were previously.

Don't panic and definitely don't give up. I was quite horrified at the state of my abdomen after my second baby—a crinkly baby elephant comes to mind. I kept with the exercise and good nutrition and it took longer the second time, but it was still improving 12–18 months later. Skin relies on elastic properties to regain shape, so gaining *and* losing weight more slowly during and after pregnancy helps prevent damage and aids a gradual return to shape. Skin is also more likely to sag if you lose weight quickly *without* exercise. If you lose fat under the skin without maintaining or increasing muscle tissue, the skin can wrinkle or sag with nothing to fill it out. Exercise also enhances circulation and therefore increases blood flow and hydration to the skin.

Look to no-one but yourself in setting goals. Don't compare your body with your sister's, your friend's or a celebrity mum's. Although all mothers essentially have a similar experience in pregnancy, we all have our own stories, we're all affected differently and there's a huge range of 'normal'. You don't often see the complete effects of motherhood on other women's bodies—only your own.

I can take a fairly good guess at what mothers of young children want; I am one, I know many and have worked with more.

The post-baby body wish list

- To lose weight and 'baby fat'.
- To 'tone up'—this means strengthen muscles.
- To achieve a shape closer to pre-pregnancy than that of a fertility statue.
- To flatten the abdomen, so you don't still look pregnant a year later—you need to rehabilitate abdominal muscles, which will also relieve back pain.
- To fit into sizes and styles of clothes you used to or want to wear.
- To increase energy—you can never have enough; this means getting fitter and increasing your metabolism.
- To relax, feel good, and have some time for you.

All these goals are possible, and the next few chapters detail an exercise program to help you achieve them. The program allows for rehabilitation after childbirth and increasing fitness at a reasonable rate. It is not extreme, but effective, and most importantly 'do-able'.

Even though getting healthier has its own intrinsic rewards, make a special point of rewarding your health goals with something that makes you feel good now and later—something tangible, fun and motivating. (Don't reward with food, unless it's a special experience like a particular restaurant you always wanted to try. The best rewards keep you focussed on your goal and enhance your path of achievement. Try some new running shoes or a workout bra (correct support is so underrated, particularly while breastfeeding), great music for exercising, a new piece of equipment like an exercise ball or weights, or a physical indulgence like a pedicure, hair colour or massage.

Or recharge your batteries with time out to relax, sleep in, read in a bubble bath, shop or do nothing while someone else takes charge of baby—this is a reward mothers deserve every week.

Action

Get clearance from your doctor to start exercise

Calculate your personal heart rate training zone using the Karvonen formula

Go for a brisk walk and try the 'talk test' to measure exercise intensity

Mark potential exercise time slots in your schedule

Make a list of exercise activities you'd like to try, then book them in

Consider equipment to help achieve your goals—start simple, with comfy clothes, appropriate shoes, a great pram or some music

Assess your fitness goals and aim for your personal best

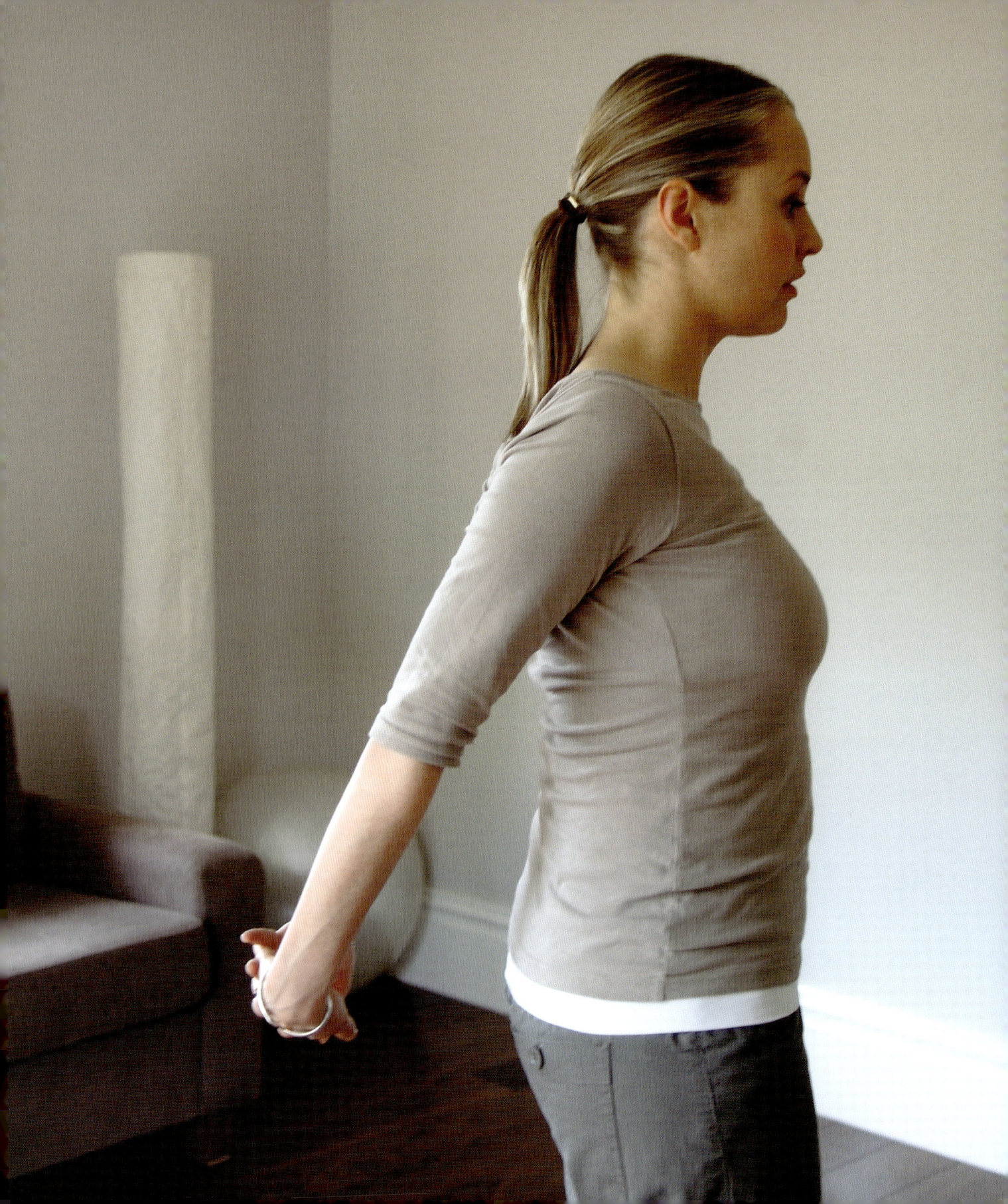

Exercising in pregnancy

I mentioned in the introduction that I was fit before getting pregnant. I was running, doing yoga, eating well—seriously fit. I was supposed to be one of those pregnant women you see power-walking or teaching fitness classes at four weeks before delivery. I knew how to keep muscle definition, to put on a healthy amount of weight and grow a cute baby belly. I wouldn't succumb to cravings for empty calories. I would exercise right up to the birth, have a drug-free experience, start exercising again soon after and snap back into shape in record time . . . I was, after all, an exercise physiologist who had been instructing others (including pregnant women) in fitness for well over a decade.

But my body decided none of this was to be. I got pregnant and the hormones took over. I had drips, drugs, immobilising sickness, debilitating pain from an enlarged corpus luteum cyst, steroid bloat, water retention, excess skin pigmentation and excessive fat gain (due to a sickness-forced 'crash diet'). I had strained pelvic floor and abdominal muscles, hip pain, back pain, swollen extremities, dislocated ribs—I could barely walk across the room in the third trimester, let alone think about a step class!

Other women experience other obstacles to fitness during pregnancy, including nausea, exhaustion, hypertension, hospitalisation for placenta praevia, treatment for pregnancy-induced diabetes, recurrent thrush (due to hormones), IVF treatment, joint and pelvic floor pain, and prescribed inactivity in the first trimester due to previous miscarriage.

So, even though I will recommend how to stay fit during pregnancy, I will be the first to understand if you don't or can't, and will be ready to guide you from the birth onwards, no matter what shape you become!

Ready?

See your doctor and get the all-clear to exercise

Exercise moderately to enjoy its many benefits

Don't forget to drink water

Keep your nutrition on track—don't blow it

Try the exercise program and track your progress

Get ready for your brand-new life

There are many benefits to both mother and baby of being in good shape before and during pregnancy. Exercise during pregnancy keeps your energy levels up, your weight gain in a healthy range, relieves stress and back pain, helps prevent gestational diabetes, constipation and varicose veins, and gives you endurance for labour and a headstart to regaining your pre-baby shape. But it is not a time to dramatically increase your fitness. There is much evidence on the safety and benefits of moderate exercise for modest fitness gains for a sedentary woman and maintenance of pre-pregnancy fitness levels for others.

All recommendations for exercise are based on the assumption of prior medical evaluation and clearance for exercise, that no contraindications exist, and that the pregnancy is considered 'normal' or without obstetric or other medical complications.

The minimum exercise recommendation for all adults is 30 minutes or more of moderate intensity physical activity on most days—if not every day—of the week. Unless otherwise advised by a doctor, a previously active and relatively fit pregnant woman can continue this. Moderate activity for an average woman equates to brisk walking at five to six kilometres per hour. You could do sessions of up to 60 minutes on most days as a maximum without requiring monitoring for extreme activity.

Previously sedentary women can begin exercising, but start with five or 10 minutes of low-intensity activity (a gentle walk) two or three days a week and gradually increase the duration, intensity and frequency. Make your goal 20–30-minute sessions three times a week.

Intensity can be measured by heart rate. It is usually recommended pregnant women keep their heart rate below 140 beats per minute during exercise. This ensures the foetus has a continual sufficient supply of oxygen and nutrients, which may otherwise be diverted to the working muscles in very intense exercise.

The type of exercise you do depends on what you were doing before pregnancy and what you enjoy. The best form of exercise for pregnant women is without doubt in the water—the benefits are many and the risks are fewer than with other forms of exercise. If you have access to a local pool, beach or aqua-fitness class, this is ideal. Water is weight-supportive and buoyancy is a great relief for the increasingly pregnant body, which often suffers back and joint pain due to the new weight carried in front. The risk of falls and sprains due to joint laxity (looser joints) is also practically non-existent and immersion in water also aids thermoregulation. Women suffering hypertension, who may otherwise be excluded from participation in exercise, can benefit from a decrease in blood pressure caused by immersion in water. Swimming and water aerobics are great workouts for any fitness level. They can be as gentle as required, but the water resistance means that even the most highly conditioned athlete can really get their heart rate up in the pool.

Walking is another great form of exercise for pregnant women as it's free and can be done anywhere. When pregnant, your workout naturally gets harder due to the increasing weight you carry (your baby). This means that if you keep it up, you get fitter and stronger as the nine months progress, even if you do the same walk every time. Women who start out very fit, however, may experience an overall decline in fitness level and should aim for maintenance. You can get a good workout walking briskly up hills or on sand, but jogging becomes less safe and less comfortable as your baby grows.

There are many other recreational and sporting pursuits which provide great exercise while pregnant, but do consider the risks to the pregnant body and baby when deciding on an activity, especially any that carries risks of falls or collisions (as in team sports, for example). As pregnancy progresses, consider changes in joint stability, balance, centre of gravity, reaction time and agility as they present increasing risks in certain activities. Your doctor should be your first point of reference in deciding about sport during pregnancy, as you are unique and no-one else's experience applies.

Strength training helps maintain lean body mass (muscle), keeps energy levels high (as muscles store glucose energy), helps the body adapt to the increasing weight of the baby and keeps you in better shape for after pregnancy. Strength or resistance training is safe during pregnancy, but relatively low weights and a higher number of repetitions are recommended. You can use just your body weight or some basic equipment for an easy workout at home. The program in this chapter includes some easy strength exercises.

Flexibility training, stretching and yoga are relaxing and provide relief for stressed mums with tight muscles. However, during pregnancy the body produces a hormone called relaxin which can increase joint laxity (looseness). This is so bones and joints can move to accommodate the growing baby and for baby's passage through the pelvis at birth. Therefore, any stretches should work through only a normal range of motion.

Stretching beyond this to increase your range of motion or performing ballistic moves (bouncing into a stretch, like dancers do) could lead to permanently loose joints. If you attend a yoga or stretch class (or any exercise class), tell the instructor you are pregnant and they will adapt the exercises for you. Or try a pregnancy yoga DVD at home. Yoga is particularly efficient as many of the poses incorporate both strength and flexibility training.

After the first trimester, pregnant women should avoid the supine position (lying on your back) during exercise and rest because the weight of the foetus impedes the return of blood to the heart.

STAY HYDRATED DURING EXERCISE

Adequate water intake is essential during pregnancy. Your blood volume increases and about one-third of the amniotic fluid is replaced each hour at some stages. During exercise, water is lost through perspiration, which is a thermoregulatory response—your body cools when sweat evaporates from the skin. So, you must be sufficiently hydrated to regulate your own and your baby's core temperatures.

It is important to replace water lost during exercise and to drink more in hot weather. To monitor this, weigh yourself immediately before and after exercise. If you lose 200 grams, for example, that means you need to drink 200 millilitres—remember, weight lost during exercise is water, not fat!

Avoid exercising in excessively hot and humid conditions. Pregnant women already have a higher basal metabolic rate (which generates more heat production), and exercise further increases body temperature. Moderate exercise in mild or temperature-controlled conditions will prevent dehydration, extreme core temperatures and excessive blood redirection away from the uterus.

NOURISH YOURSELF

A healthy attitude is essential for a healthy pregnancy. Past weight problems may cause unnecessary stress about the inevitable weight and shape changes to come. But you cannot control it all and should just focus on looking after your body by nourishing it well and keeping it fit.

Proper nutrition and exercise helps weight gain stay in the healthy range, leaving you with less to lose afterwards. Restrictive diets or

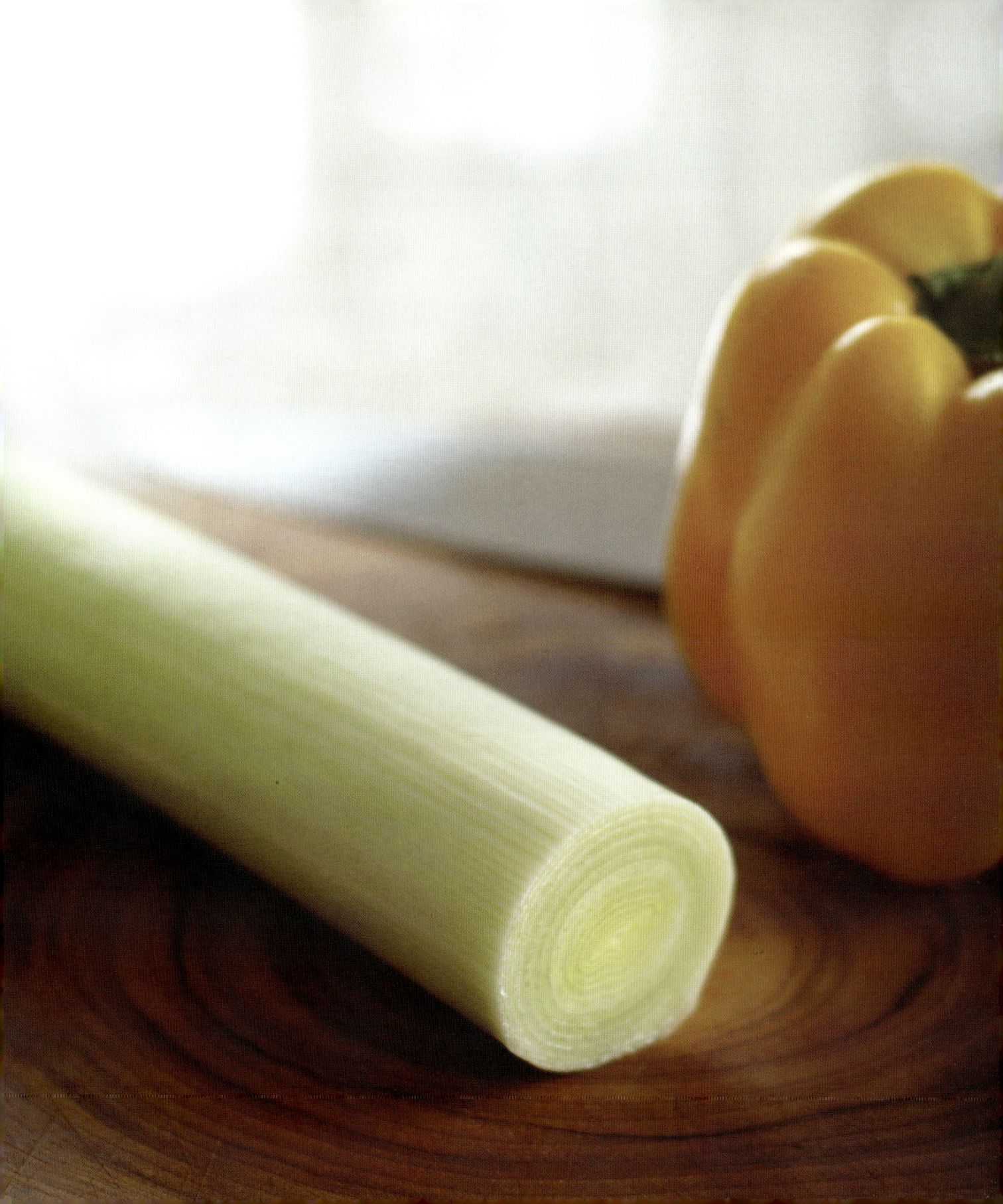

excessive exercise regimens can be dangerous for foetal development. However, excessive consumption of 'empty' calories from fats and sugars doesn't do you or baby any favours either. Research shows this type of diet increases the risk of gestational diabetes and results in babies born with more body fat.

Energy (kilojoule) requirements increase as pregnancy progresses and body weight increases, especially if you're exercising. But you don't need to eat for two—nor even for one and a half. If you do, after your baby is born, you'll still have one of you to lose! If you have not yet seen a really fresh newborn close up, at an average of three to four kilograms, they are tiny and skinny! They look nothing like cute chubby babies at a couple of months old. You don't need that much extra energy to feed babies on the inside. It actually requires more calories to breastfeed a hungry and rapidly growing infant when he's on the outside.

Ravenous appetites and cravings are common, especially in early pregnancy, but it's important to make conscious, healthy choices to satiate these or you risk slipping into poor eating habits that will be hard to break. If you crave salty foods, try rice crackers instead of chips, which are loaded with fat. If it's sugar you want, before grabbing a bag of snakes or chocolates, try fruit. Grapes, berries, peaches, sultanas or fruit yoghurt, for example, are all super-sweet with plenty of natural (not added) sugars as well as vitamins, minerals and fibre. Your health is made up of what you do 'most of the time'. So, as long as you eat well most of the time, there's no reason you can't keep your favourite treats on the menu too. If you're deprived you're more likely to give in to temptation more often. No-one expects you to be perfect, but don't live on junk food just because you think you're going to lose your figure anyway . . .

For a healthy, steady weight gain, your doctor can advise what to aim for, based on your frame size, pre-pregnancy 'extra' weight and baby weight to come.

A couple of tips for eating during pregnancy: eat when you are hungry, have breakfast before morning exercise and eat again soon after exercising. Eating more frequently in smaller amounts gives you constant energy throughout the day, as do slow-release energy foods (see chapter 5). This helps keep cravings at bay—and smaller, more frequent meals are more comfortable as the baby grows and presses on your stomach!

The nine months of pregnancy gives you plenty of time to 'nest' and prepare for the new addition. Don't forget to prepare yourself for the new job and a whole new life. This includes getting your family and home organised. If you have some 'down time' in the last trimester, use it to set yourself up for success after the baby is born. You can plan meals and a menu rotation, an exercise program and family schedules (see chapters 3, 6, and 7 for help). Then, when baby arrives with his own ever-changing schedule, at least you have priorities sorted and a framework to use. This may all sound like too much work, but whatever you put in now will save you so much more in the future.

Work on your support system. Think of people in your circle of sympathetic or like-minded friends; they are a godsend after the birth when you're wondering daily whether what your baby's doing is normal. Perhaps you have old friends, relatives or neighbours who have recently had babies. Make contact, make friends and invite them over for coffee. And don't discount the vital support you'll get from other childless friends and family members too, as they may know you best.

YOUR EXERCISE PLAN

Before starting, it is essential to get permission from your doctor as there are some contraindications to exercise during pregnancy. Then aim to walk, swim or do another appropriate aerobic activity which gets your heart rate up—like an exercise class or video—three times a week for 30 minutes.

Along with that, the following exercise program is designed to help keep you strong and flexible. It is safe to do every day, but aim for at least three times a week. All together, it should take no longer than 30 minutes—or you can break it up throughout the day.

There are many other exercises you could add, but if you keep it really simple, you're more likely to do it. Go for a walk, do a few simple exercises and some stretches while relaxing. That's it, short and sweet: no need for a long, elaborate ritual which you wouldn't get through very often.

Points to remember while exercising

- Breathe throughout exercises and stretches—don't hold your breath.
- Perform all exercises slowly, with no swinging or bouncing movements.
- Remember to stretch—review the guidelines on flexibility training in chapter 7.

TABLE 8.1 Pregnancy exercise tracker

EXERCISE/AIM	MONDAY	TUESDAY	WEDNESDAY	THURSDAY	FRIDAY	SATURDAY	SUNDAY
Walking							
Pelvic floor/ 6 sets of 10 slow and fast							
Squat/ 3 sets of 10							
Push-ups/ 3 sets of 10							
Hip rotation/10 each way							
Cat stretch/3							
Triceps & shoulder stretch/3							
Back twist/3							
Chest opener stretch/3							
Thigh stretch/3							
Inner-thigh stretch/3							
Seated toe touch/3							
Neck stretch/3							

TABLE 8.2 Pregnancy exercise tracker example

EXERCISE/AIM	MONDAY	TUESDAY	WEDNESDAY	THURSDAY	FRIDAY	SATURDAY	SUNDAY
Walking	20 mins	10 mins x 2		15 mins		35 mins	
Pelvic floor/ 6 sets of 10 slow and fast	X	X	X	X	X	X	X
Squat/ 3 sets of 10	10/8/5		10/9/5				
Push-ups/ 3 sets of 10	5/5		6/6/5				
Hip rotation /10 each way	X	X					
Cat stretch /3	X	X	X		X		
Triceps & shoulder stretch/3	X		X			X	
Back twist /3	X	X				X	X
Chest opener stretch /3	X		X		X		
Thigh stretch /3	X				X		
Inner-thigh stretch /3	X	X			X		
Seated toe touch /3	X	X			X		X
Neck stretch /3	X	X					X

Notes: Try to walk and do pelvic floor exercises every day and the other exercises at least three times a week.
Record the number of repetitions and sets; for example, 10/10/8 means you did three sets of the exercise, first 10 times, then 10 again and then 8 in the final set.

- Do not strain or push too hard—these exercises should be relatively easy to do several times over.
- If you feel faint or dizzy, stop, rest and try again some other time.
- If anything hurts, or if you get any cramping or bleeding, stop and consult your doctor.
- Listen to your body; if you're tired, rest.
- Sip water as needed.
- Relax and enjoy—it's not hard, and you'll feel good afterwards!

An exercise program tracker is included (see table: 8.1) to help you track your progress, along with an example (see table 8.2 and Chapter 9 on sets and reps for how to fill it out) of how to fill it out. You can copy the program chart for as many weeks as you need, and then simply check off the exercises as you do them.

PELVIC FLOOR EXERCISES

Performing pelvic floor exercises during pregnancy will keep these muscles working well and aid a speedier recovery after the birth (see chapter 9).

SQUATS (Photo 8.1)

These are easy to do, and a great all-round lower body exercise.
- Stand with your feet about shoulder-width apart.
- Keeping your knees above your feet, bend your knees and squat into a sitting position, really sticking your backside out behind you. Raising your arms to the front while you squat helps you balance, especially as the tummy gets bigger, or you can stand next to a chair or wall for balance.
- Imagine there is a small chair behind you and you are sitting on it. Your knees should not bend forward past the toes. Bend knees no more than 90 degrees, and aim for thighs parallel to the ground.

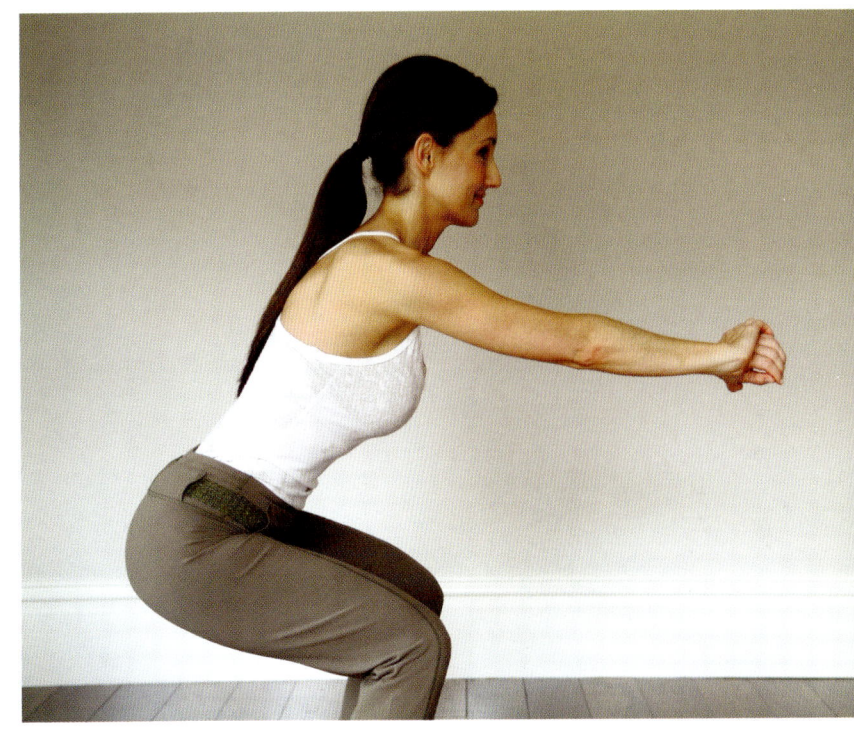

Photo 8.1 Squats

EXERCISING IN PREGNANCY 145

PUSH-UPS

These support the breasts and shape the arms. They're better for you than you think and not as hard as they look. Perform all variations slowly and under control.

LEVEL 1: WALL PUSH-UP (Photo 8.2)

- ❖ Face a wall, standing about 30 cm away. Place your hands on the wall at shoulder height, a little wider than shoulder-width apart, fingers angled in slightly.
- ❖ Bending your elbows out to the sides, slowly take your chest towards the wall. Then push away, back to your starting position. If it's too easy, stand further away from the wall.
- ❖ Breathing technique: inhale going into the wall, exhale pushing out.

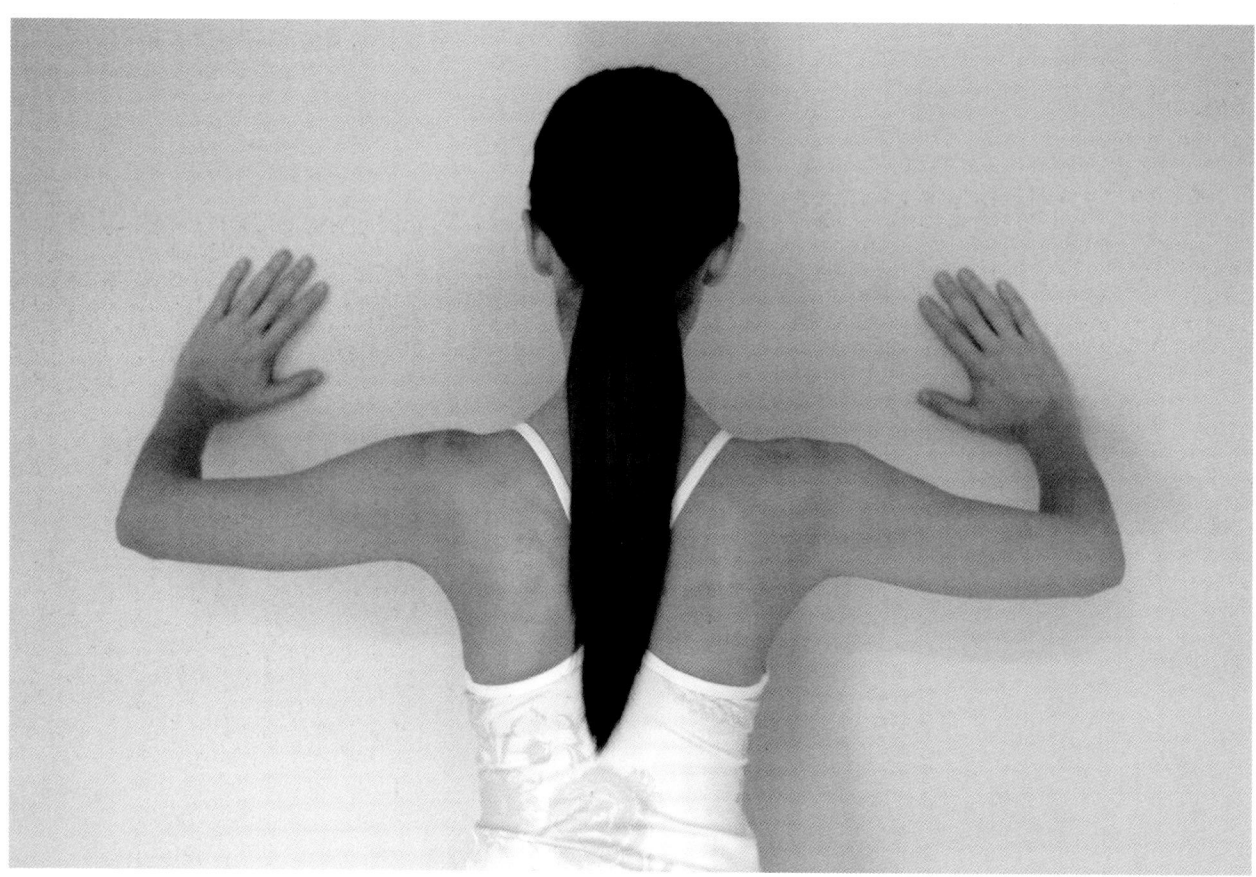

Photo 8.2 Wall Push-ups

LEVEL 2: PRINCESS PUSH-UP (Photo 8.3)

- Start on your hands and knees, with your hands under your shoulders and fingers angled in slightly. Brace your mid-section if you can to support your back. Keep your back and neck straight and look at the ground.
- Lower your chest towards the floor, bending your elbows out to the sides, then push back up.
- When you can do three sets of 10 repetitions (30 in total), gradually take more weight onto your hands by walking them further away from your knees (see Photo 9.6). Remember to keep your back straight (no 'sway back').
- Breathing technique: inhale going down, exhale pushing up.

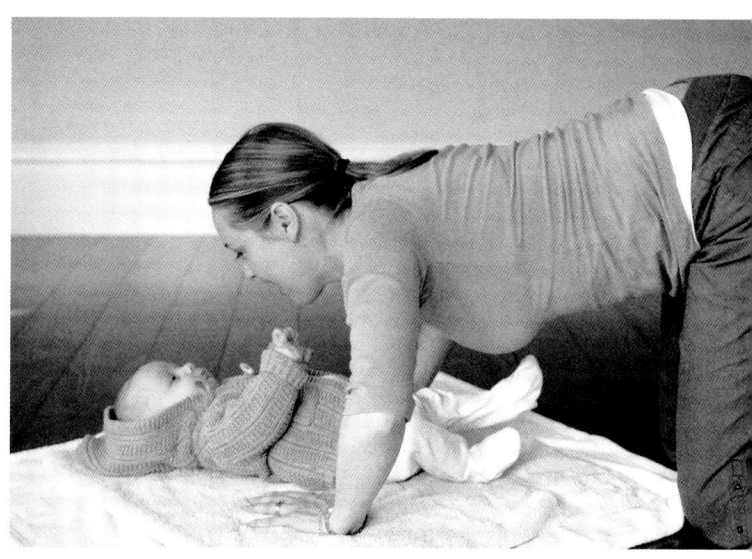

Photo 8.3 Princess Push-ups

HIP ROTATION (Photo 8.4)

- Sitting, balancing or rotating on an exercise ball is good for stability and strength of core muscles and relieves a tight lower back. No ball? No worries, do it standing.
- Sit on the ball and rotate your hips slowly in one direction, then go the other way. Do 10 circles each way.
- To do it standing, start with your feet shoulder-width apart and knees slightly bent. Rotate your hips around slowly in an exaggerated hula-hoop movement. Do it both ways.

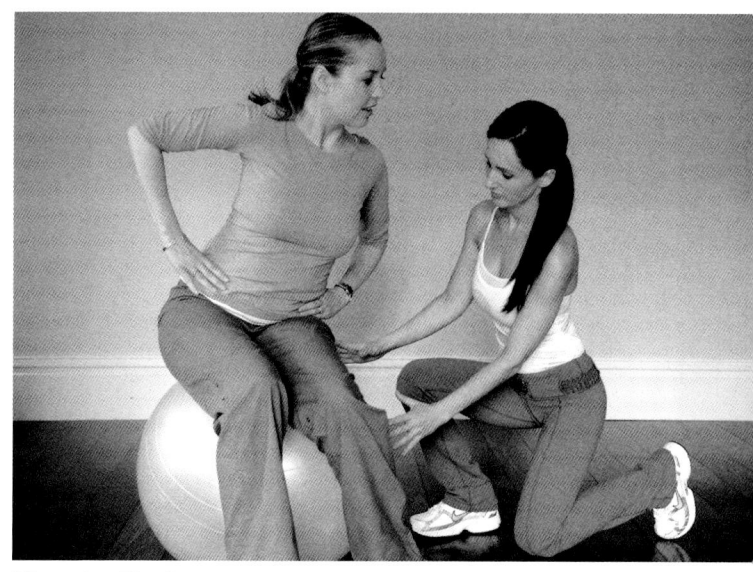

Photo 8.4 Hip Rotation

CAT STRETCH (Photo 8.5)

This helps relieve back muscles which tighten during pregnancy to support the growing belly.

- Get down on your hands and knees. Arch your back, curl your tummy in and drop your head down. Tuck your hips under, stretching the lower back and round through the upper back, stretching between shoulders.
- Hold and breathe. Relax to a flat back and repeat.

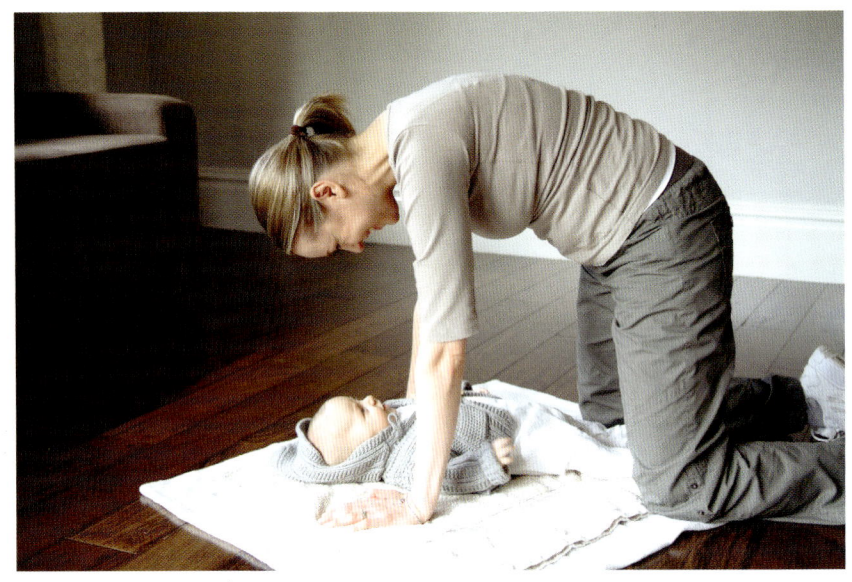

Photo 8.5 Cat Stretch

TRICEPS AND SHOULDER STRETCH

The aim is to hold your hands behind your back—don't forget to change sides.

- Holding a towel in one hand, take your arm up over your head and bend your elbow behind your head.
- Reach your other hand up your back to grab the towel. Walk the hands together along the towel and hold when you can't go any further. (See Photo 9.10)

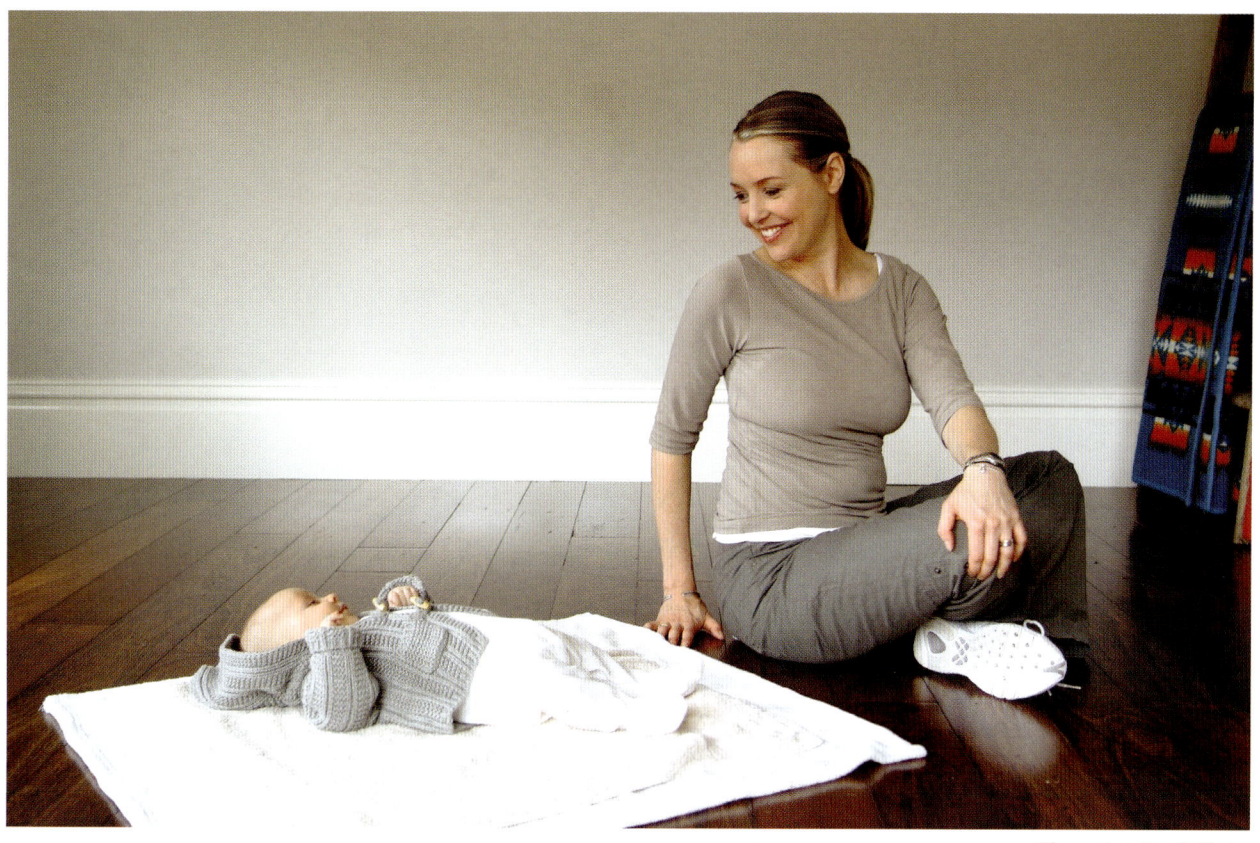

Photo 8.6 Back Twist

BACK TWIST (Photo 8.6)

Most pregnant women experience backaches as abdominal muscles no longer support the spine effectively. This stretch helps relieve pressure on the spine.

- ❖ Sit on the floor, legs crossed. Twist around to the right to look behind you and place your left hand on your right thigh. Hold, relax your back and breathe. Change sides.

CHEST OPENER STRETCH

This exercise stretches the front of the shoulders, arms and chest.
- ❖ Clasp hands behind your back, then pull back and up to lift your arms—do not lean forward or shrug shoulders. Hold.
  (See Photo 9.2)

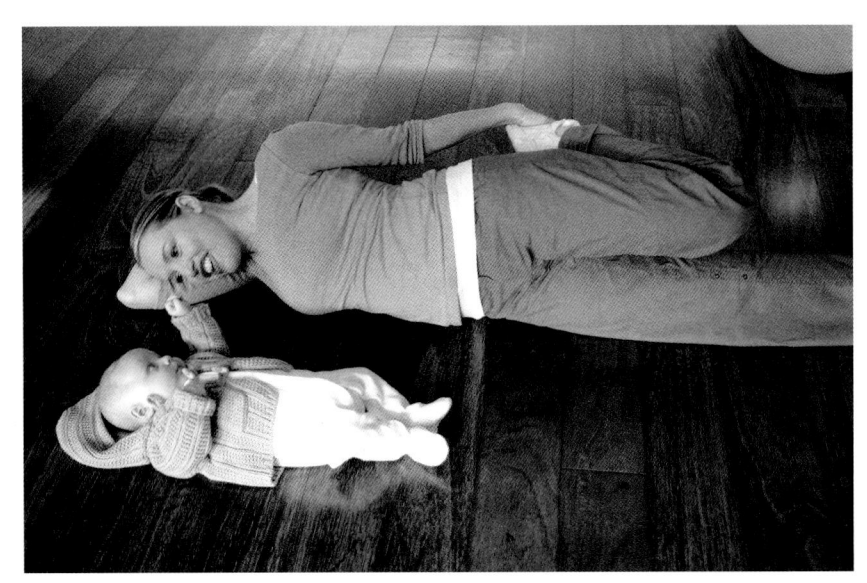

Photo 8.7 Thigh Stretch

THIGH STRETCH (PHOTO 8.7)
You should feel this stretch on the front of the thigh and hip.
- ❖ Lie on your right side, with your body in a straight line—support your belly with a pillow if necessary. Rest your head on your right arm.
- ❖ Keeping your knees together, bend your left knee (the leg on top) and pull the left heel into the buttocks with your left hand. Repeat on the other side.

INNER-THIGH STRETCH (PHOTO 8.8)
Take care not to round through the back. Just sitting in the starting position is usually enough of a stretch for most women.
- ❖ Sit on the floor and stretch your legs out to the sides. Try to keep your legs straight.
- ❖ Place your hands on the floor in front of you and sit up as straight as you can.
- ❖ Bending through the hip joint, lean forward with a straight back and walk your hands forward as you go. Stop when you feel the stretch.

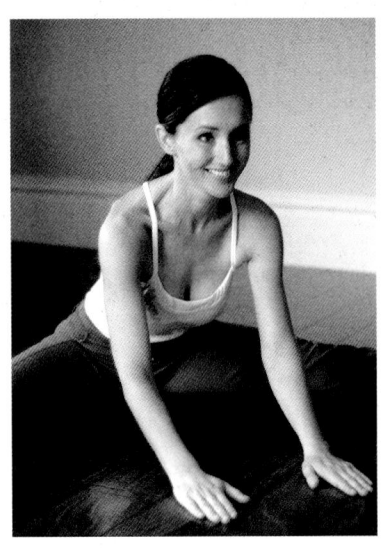

Photo 8.8 Inner-thigh Stretch

SEATED TOE TOUCH

This stretches the lower back and hamstring muscles (back of the thigh), which get tight when you sit a lot.

- Sit on the ground with your legs together, stretched out in front. Reach forward and try to touch your toes, relaxing and rounding through the back. Try to keep your knees straight.
- To increase the stretch, use a towel. Take one end in each hand and hook it over your feet to pull into a deeper stretch. (See Photo 9.4)

NECK STRETCH (PHOTO 8.9)

The neck and shoulders feel the strain of supporting growing breasts. This stretch brings relief and helps prevent headaches.

- Drop your head to one side, to feel a stretch down the other side of the neck. To increase the stretch, put your hand on the side of your head and gently pull your head down further towards the shoulder. Hold.
- Change sides by slowly rolling the head to the front and to the other side, feeling the stretch down the back of the neck.

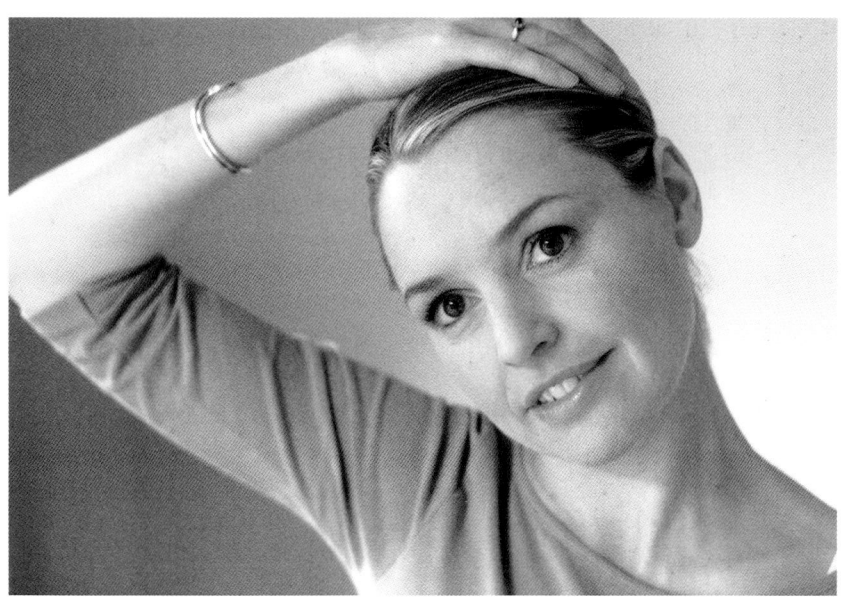

Photo 8.9 Neck Stretch

Action

Check with your doctor that it's okay for you to exercise, then start today

Look at your eating habits—be realistic, can you improve?

Have regular health checks before and during pregnancy

Start collecting favourite recipes— healthy and fast or freezer-friendly

Share your excitement and experience with friends, family and other mums

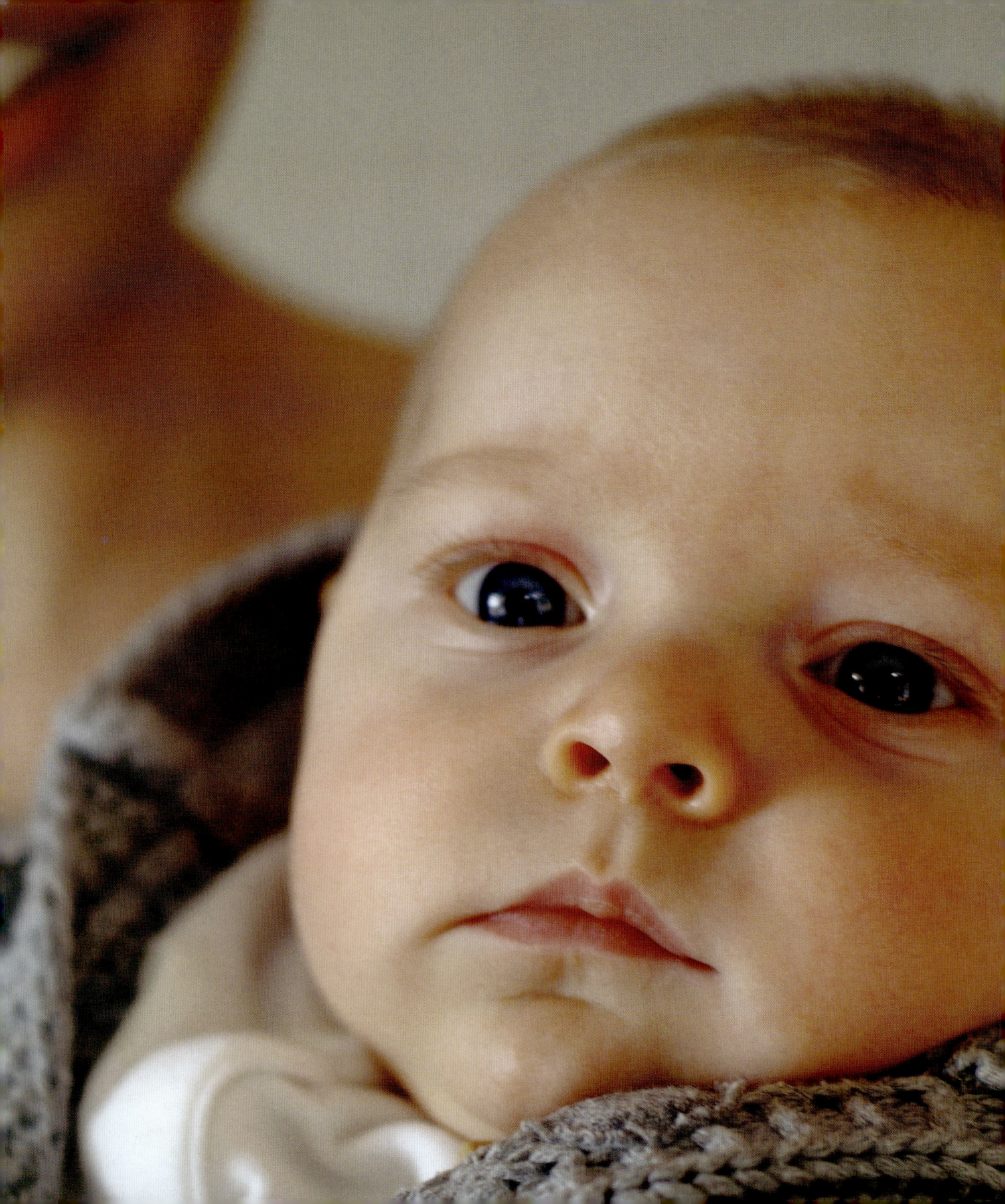

The first trimester after birth

When you've just had a baby, the first priority is to take it easy. While you're in hospital, use the experts on hand and learn as much as you can—not only about baby, but also what's going on with you. When you get home, get as much rest as possible, particularly if you have extra help in the first couple of weeks. Caring for your first baby is a steep learning curve, but don't neglect your own needs. Have plenty of fresh fruit, vegies and water, and nap when baby does. Don't try to do it all—relax, enjoy this special time to bond with your baby and let others help you around the house, with meals and with other children.

You can feel like a big milking cow if you sit around feeding and tending to an infant all day. Exercise helps fight fatigue and lethargy, so you can feel more like a racehorse than a cow. It also helps with 'baby blues', which often accompany hormone changes after the birth.

As each three-month trimester of pregnancy has distinct developmental phases for you and baby, I like to use three-month trimesters *after* birth to mark phases of recovery and improving fitness. Your plan is to get back in shape in the same amount of time it took to get out of it. It's fair and realistic . . . but don't worry, there's also a Plan B.

KEEPING IT SIMPLE

My exercise sections are among the shortest in the book. I could give you a huge collection of elaborate exercises from which to choose and build a two-hour daily routine of cardio work and exercises to strengthen

Ready?

What you can do within 24 hours of giving birth

Exercises to aid recovery over the first six weeks

Getting the pelvic floor back in shape

Proper abdominal training after babies— no gadgets required

After your check-up, step it up to see real results

Exercise programs to follow and track your progress

and stretch every inch of your body from the day the baby's born. But you won't do it and neither would I, because we live in the real world.

Time is precious and by keeping it as simple as possible you're set up for success. If you do more exercise than I recommend, excellent! But I want you to start in a way that gently works the exercise habit into your new lifestyle and lets you recognise the benefits.

For the first three months after the birth, I've chosen the best all-round exercises to address immediate muscular concerns after delivery, raise your fitness level, relieve pain and set you up for some real body work to come.

I haven't included any equipment in the initial nine-month exercise programs—no bands, no balls, no gadgets. Although your workouts may be more challenging with basic weights or a ball, you can get back in shape just with your body. Mothers have so many baby accessories to buy, organise and carry around that a range of fitness accessories is last on the list—needing equipment could just become one more excuse for not exercising. Chapter 12 has a program using equipment, which you can progress to when you're ready—whether that's six months or two years after a birth.

You don't have to do all exercises in one session, not even the walking. You can break it up and spread it throughout the day. For example, do two 15-minute walks instead of one 30-minute walk and do your strength and stretching exercises while baby sleeps, has 'tummy time' on a rug or watches from a rocker. You can fit in a set of squats while watching the news or waiting for the kettle to boil. You don't need to start off doing it all. Work up to the recommended number of repetitions for each exercise in the program. Prioritising it is the key. Keep the exercise trackers handy to remind you, and record and watch your progress over the weeks.

And remember, if there's ever any pain, cramping or extra bleeding while exercising in the first three months after giving birth, stop and see your doctor.

HOW TO USE THE EXERCISE TRACKER

Each exercise program is presented in a table for you to track your exercise. You can copy the program pages for as many weeks as you need, and then simply check off the exercises as you do them.

Sets and reps

Some of the programs have more detail, where you can record how many sets and repetitions you perform. A 'repetition' (or 'rep' in gym speak) is doing an exercise once. You perform several repetitions in a row in what is called a 'set', then have a short rest to let muscles recover before doing another set. By tracking this information you'll know when it's time to move on to a harder exercise or heavier weight.

When you have been able to do the prescribed number of sets and repetitions (or even more) for a couple of weeks, you need to make it harder so that you get stronger and fitter. With some exercises like push-ups, when you get to the hardest version—push-ups on the toes—and you can do three sets of 20, you may want to just keep doing this for maintenance, or you can start lifting weights and move on to a bench press.

Some exercise experts recommend three sets for weight training, others recommend two sets. If you always have limited time, I'd rather you get in two sets of everything than do the first couple of exercises, run out of time and habitually skip the rest.

This exercise plan is very different to a 'body-building' program and it is relatively fast and easy. A great way to speed up your workout is to alternate or rotate between a few exercises and keep moving. Instead of resting, change to a different exercise which uses different muscles. You'll still rest each muscle group between sets, but you'll keep moving, get your heart rate up more and spend less total time exercising. You can also use the time between sets to stretch the muscles you're working, which also saves time.

THE FIRST 24 HOURS: YOUR EXERCISE PLAN

If you did not have a caesarean birth or any major complications, your doctor or midwife will probably encourage you to start walking around soon after delivery. Walking aids your recovery and improves circulation and strengthens pelvic floor and torso muscles.

You can potentially start strengthening your pelvic floor and abdominal muscles within hours of giving birth. This depends on two things: clearance from your doctor and how you feel. Your doctor will advise you on issues such as stitches, abdominal separation, high blood pressure, gestational diabetes or risk of prolapsed uterus. Exercise may be the last thing on your mind, but the pelvic floor needs rehabilitation, and not doing this can lead to complications such as incontinence and a prolapsed uterus.

Pelvic floor exercises

Prenatal books and classes always include exercises for the pelvic floor, so hopefully you'll have learned these by the time you give birth. Pregnancy puts a lot of stress on the pelvic floor. There's the weight of the baby and also hormones relaxing your ligaments preparing for baby to travel down the birth canal. So even if you had a caesarean, these muscles have weakened, which is not news to you if you were unlucky enough to contract a cough or cold in your third trimester.

The layers of muscles which support the uterus, bladder and bowel make up the floor or base of the pelvis and stretch like a hammock from the tail bone in the back to the pubic bone in front. Rehabilitation of these muscles should start as soon as possible after birth. If you don't want to be left in nappies after your children are toilet trained, get squeezing!

IDENTIFYING THE PELVIC FLOOR MUSCLES

It is easiest (and safest) to do this on the toilet after giving birth.

- Tighten the muscles around the anus as though preventing passing wind, keep the buttocks relaxed, then release.
- When you urinate, stop the flow by squeezing the muscles around the urethra. This should only be done initially to identify the muscles then occasionally to check your progress, but not on a regular basis as it can interfere with normal bladder function.
- Once you have identified these muscles at the base of the pelvis, try contracting them all together from the tail bone through to the pubic bone. Keep abdominal and buttock muscles relaxed and breathe normally. It should feel like 'pulling up' the area, then letting it go. It may not feel like much of a squeeze at first—all the more reason to do it.

LEVEL 1

Squeeze the muscles and hold for five seconds. Rest for 10 seconds and repeat. Do as many as you can and work up to Level 2.

LEVEL 2: THE 'TENS'

- 10 contractions
- 10-second hold
- 10-second rest between each
- 10 short, fast, strong squeezes, to finish.

The short, fast, stronger contractions are for extra support for sudden increases of pressure on the pelvic floor, such as when you cough, sneeze, jump or lift.

You can do your 'tens' anytime, anywhere—in the car, on the phone, eating breakfast, brushing your teeth, lying in bed, feeding baby. Do them whenever you remember: the more you do, the stronger they'll become. But as a minimum, do them at every feed, so you should get at least six sets a day.

You should really never stop doing pelvic floor exercises after you have a baby. Multiple pregnancies, weight gain and menopause all weaken the pelvic floor, so this is a habit to adopt for life. It really pays off in terms of freedom and independence in the short and long term.

If you have trouble identifying or exercising these muscles, ask your doctor for help. No matter how embarrassing you may find it now, it'll be much more embarrassing later if you don't!

Abdominal exercises

Weak abdominal muscles increase the risk of injury and pain in the lower back and can leave you looking pregnant long after you have a baby. An abdominal separation (diastasis) is common after pregnancy. It is where the more superficial abdominal muscle—the rectus abdominis ('six-pack' muscle)—has separated down the middle to accommodate the growing belly. To check for diastasis, lie on your back and gently lift your head off the floor. Feel the area directly above your navel, where you may feel a hole. If it is wider than two fingers you may need extra support while the muscles heal.

It is important to change body positions carefully after having a baby. When sitting up from a lying position (such as getting out of bed), first roll onto your side and push up with your arms. Similarly, when lying down, go sideways. This prevents a 'jack-knife' position which strains the rectus abdominis muscle and can worsen a separation which has not yet healed.

These muscles should not be targeted for exercise until the separation has closed, as this can also make it worse. In some women the gap in the rectus abdominis never fully closes, but give it time and help it by strengthening the deeper abdominal (core) muscles. So forget the crunches for now and stick to the core.

The transversus abdominis (or the transverse abdominal) is a deep core muscle which provides postural support. It wraps horizontally around the body like a thick belt worn by competitive weightlifters and it supports the spine. It is connected to the more superficial rectus abdominis at the front, so you can pull in your whole tummy by contracting the transverse muscle, which is the best way to encourage a separation to heal. Much lower back pain is associated with a weak transverse abdominal, particularly after pregnancy. Strengthening this muscle not only saves your back but also gives you a waistline again, rather than an apple-shaped torso which can persist.

You can start exercising the transverse abdominal as soon as your doctor gives you the nod after birth. It is a relief to finally sit or stand with support after months of a heavy weight literally hanging off the front of your body.

IDENTIFYING THE TRANSVERSE ABDOMINAL

- Lie on your back and place one hand over your belly button.
- Inhale, then as you exhale pull your belly button back in towards your spine, as though you're pulling your tummy in for a photo.
- Hold your tummy in and keep breathing.
- You should be able to do this with a neutral spine position; not pushing the lower back into the floor or arching it. Nothing should move, except around the waist.

LEVEL 1

Lying on your back, hold 10 contractions (as described in identifying the transverse abdominal) for 10 seconds, with a short rest in between. Tighten and increase the strength on each contraction. Remember to exhale as you pull your tummy in and keep breathing as you hold. Do at least four sets a day at feed times, along with the pelvic floor exercises.

LEVEL 2

Change to a sitting or standing position and do the same contractions as Level 1.

LEVEL 3

Get down on your hands and knees, keep a flat back and pull your tummy in and up towards your spine—you should not end up in an arched 'cat stretch' position. Hold the contraction and keep breathing.

These are difficult directly after the birth, but they get easier. Like the pelvic floor exercises, they can be done any time. Consciously contract this muscle to protect your back when you feed, lift baby, stand up, sit down or walk. When standing, be aware of your posture and hold in your tummy.

THE FIRST SIX WEEKS: YOUR EXERCISE PLAN

Start some light walking in the first three weeks. When you feel up to it, put baby in the pram or pouch and head out the door. A stroll around the block for fresh air is relaxing and relieving. It doesn't have to be far or long—that will come later—but getting out the door and realising a short walk is no big deal promotes the right attitude for getting back in shape. Chances are, you and baby will enjoy it and before long make it a daily habit.

From three to six weeks after the birth, aim for an easy walk most days and work up to 30 minutes—if you only do it every second day, that's fine! Just get moving to fight fatigue and start shifting weight.

The stretches help relieve inevitable back and shoulder tightness from holding a baby for what seems like all day and night.

Exercise tracker

Here is your exercise tracker for this stage, and an example showing how to use it. Aim to do all the exercises as frequently as possible, daily if you can. Remember, the following plan is ideal; your world is real.

TABLE 9.1 The first six weeks

EXERCISE/AIM	MONDAY	TUESDAY	WEDNESDAY	THURSDAY	FRIDAY	SATURDAY	SUNDAY
Walk / 30 mins total							
Pelvic floor/ 6 sets of 10 slow and 10 fast							
Transverse abdominal/ 6 sets of 10							
Shoulder rolls/ 10 forward and back							
Chest opener/ 3 times							
Arm crossover/ 3 each side							
Neck stretch/ 3 each side							
Seated toe touch/ 3 times							
Lower back/ 3 times							
How do you feel?							

TABLE 9.2 Example of the first six weeks

EXERCISE/AIM	MONDAY	TUESDAY	WEDNESDAY	THURSDAY	FRIDAY	SATURDAY	SUNDAY
Walk / 30 mins total	20 mins, 9 a.m.	10 mins, 9 a.m. 20 mins, 4 p.m.		30 mins, 9.30 a.m.	45 min stroll	10 mins, 11 a.m. 10 mins, 6 p.m.	
Pelvic floor / 6 sets of 10 slow and 10 fast	6 sets	6 sets	6 sets	6 sets	6 sets	6 sets	6 sets
Transverse abdominal / 6 sets of 10	4 sets	4 sets	4 sets	4 sets	4 sets	4 sets	4 sets
Shoulder rolls / 10 forward and back	X	X	X	X		X	
Chest opener / 3 times	X	X		X	X	X	
Arm crossover / 3 each side	X	X		X	X	X	
Neck stretch / 3 each side	X	X		X	X	X	
Seated toe touch / 3 times	X	X		X		X	X
Lower back / 3 times	X	X	X	X		X	
How do you feel?	Tired	Afternoon nap, nice!	Very fussy baby today	Better today, walk was nice	Walked around shops	Tired, not much sleep	Busy social day

Stamina

Start light walking—up to 30-minute sessions, or a few shorter walks—as many days as you can.

After walking, stretch your calf muscles (down the back of your lower leg): stand on the edge of a kerb or step, and gently drop one heel at a time off the back until you feel a stretch.

Also stretch the front of your thigh (quadriceps muscles). Stand on one leg, then pull the other foot in towards your buttocks, heel first, with your hand. Keep your knees together and stand up straight. Hold onto the pram for balance. (See Photo 9.1)

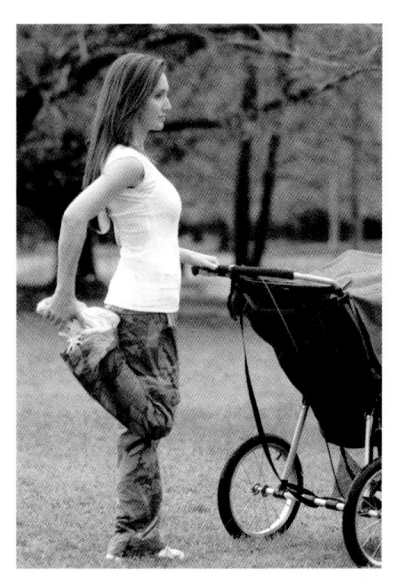

Photo 9.1 Thigh Stretch

Strength

Continue with the pelvic floor and transverse abdominal exercises daily if you can.

Walking is weight-bearing exercise which strengthens the legs and torso.

Stretch

Look back over the flexibility guidelines in chapter 7 for good technique. Always start with your spine in a neutral position and don't arch your back as you stretch; keep the abdominals tight.

Remember, don't work beyond a normal range of motion or try to increase flexibility. Just hold where you can feel the muscles gently stretching.

SHOULDER ROLLS
- Slowly roll both shoulders backwards 10 times in a large exaggerated motion. Repeat forwards.

CHEST OPENER (Photo 9.2)
- Clasp your hands behind your back, then pull back and up to lift your arms. Hold. Do not lean forward or shrug your shoulders.

Photo 9.2 Chest opener

ARM CROSSOVER (Photo 9.3)
- Keeping your shoulders down, cross one arm in front of your chest. Take your other hand and place it above the elbow of the arm you're stretching and pull it in until you feel a stretch in the back of the shoulder.

NECK STRETCH
- Drop your head to one side, to feel a stretch down the other side of the neck. To increase the stretch, put the hand on the side of your head to gently pull your head down further towards the shoulder. Hold.
- Change sides by slowly rolling the head to the front and to the other side, feeling the stretch down the back of the neck. (See photo 8.9.)

SEATED TOE TOUCH (Photo 9.4)
- Sit on the ground with your legs together, stretched out in front. Reach forward and try to touch your toes, relaxing and rounding through the back. Try to keep your knees straight.
- To increase the stretch, use a towel. Grab one end in each hand and hook it over your feet to pull into a deeper stretch. This stretches the lower back and hamstring muscles (back of the thigh) which get tight when you sit a lot.

LOWER BACK STRETCH (Photo 9.5)
- Lie on your back with your knees up and your feet flat on the floor. Contract the transverse abdominal, then push your lower back into the floor and hold.
- To increase the stretch, pull your knees in and hug them to your chest, rounding and relaxing through the spine.
- Release and stretch legs out. Repeat three times.

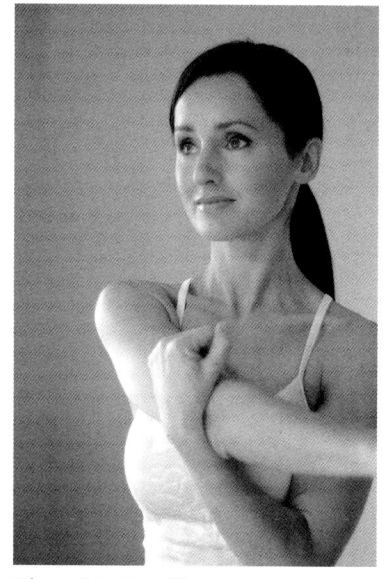

Photo 9.3 Arm Crossover

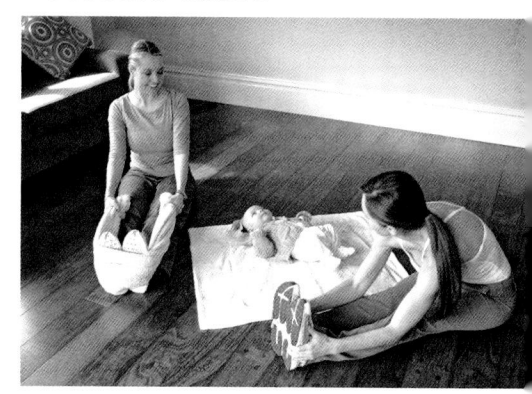

Photo 9.4 Seated Toe Touch

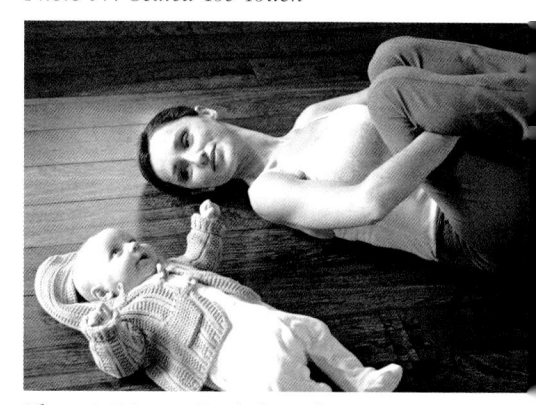

Photo 9.5 Lower Back Stretch

Scheduling

Aim to complete this exercise schedule daily, particularly the pelvic floor and abdominal exercises and stretches. By using cues as part of your new routine you can sneak in some exercise without making a big effort. And you'll create an exercise habit on which you can easily build. Try these cues for scheduling your exercise:

- **Feed times:** do pelvic floor and transverse abdominal exercises.
- **Putting baby to bed:** stretch immediately afterwards, every time you settle baby. It only takes a few minutes to feel the benefits.
- **Baby's fussy times:** instead of carrying baby around rocking or jiggling, or rolling the pram back and forth, go for a short walk with baby in a pram or pouch.

And that's it! You *can* fit some exercise into your day as a new mum. The whole program won't take long and is safe and effective for the first six weeks. If you're planning to bounce back into shape in record time, be patient. The walking and eating really help, but it's better to wait until after your six-week check-up for the more strenuous exercises in the next section. The rule is start gently (as you can always make it harder)—but first do no harm.

WEEKS SIX TO 12: YOUR EXERCISE PLAN

As the blur of the first six weeks settles down, it's now reasonable to plan a regular schedule for your exercise. Even if your baby doesn't have regular feeding and sleeping times yet, if you wait until things get more predictable, you may be waiting forever! So make realistic plans, stay flexible and have a Plan B. Baby won't cooperate with your walking schedule every time, but doing it *most* of the time is what counts.

After your six-week check-up and permission from your doctor, it's time to start a real exercise program which gives you the results you want, keeping in mind you are still healing. A walking-based program is the easiest to do with a young baby and maybe a toddler along for the ride in a double pram. If you have too many children to push, find times when someone can mind the children and you can walk alone or just with the baby—for example, when your partner's around, when other children are at preschool, or take turns minding toddlers with a friend.

Plan to walk daily—it's what our bodies are built for—but do it at least four days a week. If walking is not for you, pull out that list of activities to challenge your body, but make sure you do something that gets your heart rate up and uses a decent amount of energy.

Exercise tracker

Here is your exercise tracker for this stage with the number of sets and reps to aim for. Try to walk and do pelvic floor, transverse abs and stretch exercises daily, and strength exercises three times a week.

TABLE 9.3 Weeks six to 12

EXERCISE/AIM	SETS	REPS	MONDAY	TUESDAY	WEDNESDAY	THURSDAY	FRIDAY	SATURDAY	SUNDAY
Walk / 30 min									
Pelvic floor/ slow and fast	6	10 each							
Transverse abs	6	10							
Push up	3	10							
Crunch	3	10							
Squats	3	10							
Back extension	2	10							
Arm crossover	3								
Neck stretch	3								
Seated toe touch	3								
Lower back stretch	3								
Chest opener	3								
Triceps & shoulder stretch	3								

Stamina

Walk for 30 minutes a day—get faster, go further and try hills. This can be broken into two or three shorter walks, or substitute with another cardiovascular activity.

Strength

PUSH-UPS

As explained in chapter 8, these support the breasts and shape the arms. Perform all variations slowly and under control.

LEVEL 1: WALL PUSH-UP

- Face a wall, standing about 30 cm away. Place your hands on the wall at shoulder height, a little wider than shoulder-width apart, fingers angled in slightly.
- Keeping your abdominals pulled in, bring your chest towards the wall, bending your elbows out to the sides. Slowly push away from the wall, back to your starting position. If it's too easy,stand further away from the wall.
- Breathing technique: inhale going into the wall, exhale pushing out. (See Photo 8.2)

LEVEL 2: PRINCESS PUSH-UP

- Start on your hands and knees, with your hands under your shoulders and fingers angled in slightly. Exhale and tighten the transverse abdominal, pulling your belly button in towards the spine and keeping it there throughout the exercise. Keep your back and neck straight and look at the ground.
- Lower your chest towards the floor, bending your elbows out to the sides, then push back up. This may be easy, but start with good form and work up to three sets of 10 repetitions (30 in total). (See photo 8.3.)
- As you get stronger, take more weight onto your hands by walking them further away from your knees, until you are pushing up with a straight hip joint—that is, knees, hips and shoulders all in a straight line. But keep the tummy pulled in tightly (no 'sway back'). (See Photo 9.6)
- Breathing technique: inhale going down, exhale pushing up.

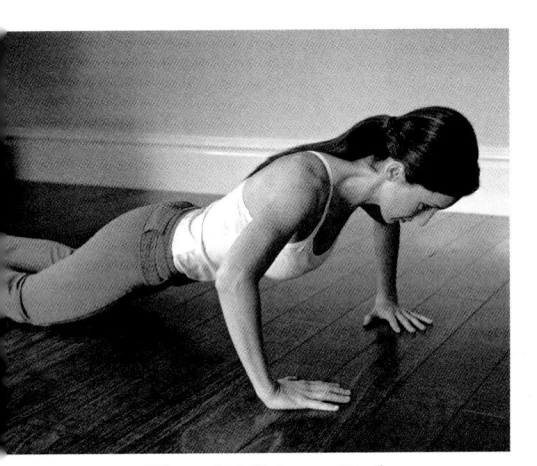

Photo 9.6 Princess Push-up

ABDOMINAL CRUNCHES (Photo 9.7)

At your six-week check-up, ask about your abdominal separation if you have one. If the muscles are still too far apart, continue the transverse abdominal exercises. Otherwise, if you are ready, you can now work the rectus abdominis and obliques—superficial muscles located at the front of the abdomen, attached to the ribs, hip bones and pubic bone.

Abdominal crunch exercises on the floor are the first place to start. An exercise ball is great for core training, but if you weren't using one during pregnancy, you need to work up to it—it is harder to crunch on a ball than on the floor, as the ball provides an unstable base.

I recommend starting on the floor to ensure good form, that any diastasis is on the mend and your muscles are strong enough before progressing. See the next chapter for abdominal training on the ball.

LEVEL 1

This exercise should feel as though you're squeezing the bottom ribs towards the hip bones. It's not about sitting up; it's about curling the torso.

- Lie on your back, knees up, feet on the floor. First, contract the transverse abdominal and keep it pulled in during this exercise—it sounds tricky, but it just takes practice. Keep your neck straight and look up at the ceiling.
- Slowly lift your head off the floor with your arms beside the body and your hands sliding towards your feet. Lift until your shoulder blades come off the floor. Count four seconds going each way, with a pause at the top.
- Breathing technique: exhale as you lift, inhale going down.

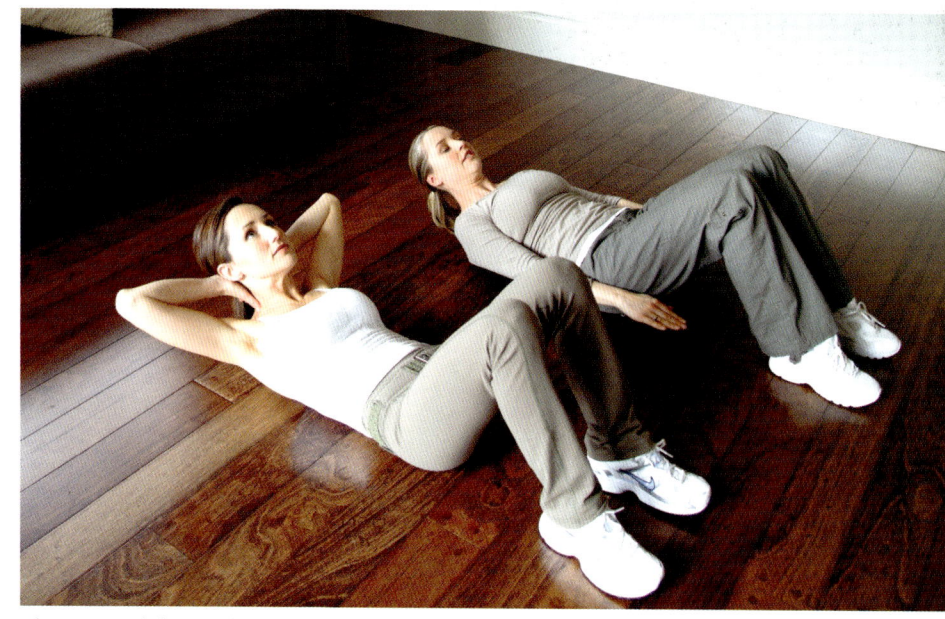

Photo 9.7 Abdominal Crunches

THE FIRST TRIMESTER AFTER BIRTH

LEVEL 2

Remember, don't do this exercise with a wide diastasis, as you risk pulling the muscles further apart if you start too early. If in doubt, leave it out. A trim waist after baby is achieved through a combination of transverse abdominal exercises, the cardio work and appropriate nutrition—*not* with hundreds of crunches.

- Place one or both hands at the base of the skull to support your head. Lay your elbows out to the sides. This provides support, but makes the crunch a little harder.
- Perform the crunch as in Level 1, but only use the hands for support—don't pull the head up; keep your neck straight and your elbows to the sides. Keep the focus on curling the torso, not the neck.

SQUATS

Do the same squat from chapter 8 in the prenatal exercise section. The slower you go, the harder it is, so challenge yourself and go really slowly—and hold those transverse abdominals in. (See photo 8.1.)

BACK EXTENSION (Photo 9.8)

This balances the exercises for the front of the body.

LEVEL 1

- Lie face-down on the floor, on a towel, mat or carpet. You can use a pillow lengthways under your torso if it is uncomfortable—or do it on a bed for ultimate comfort.
- Rest your head comfortably on your hands. Slowly lift one leg off the floor behind you, give it a good squeeze at the top, then place it down. Alternate legs.
- Breathing technique: exhale as you lift, inhale going down.
- The areas you should feel tightening are the back of the thigh, the buttocks and the lower back. When you can do three sets of 20 repetitions on each leg, move to Level 2.

LEVEL 2

- ❖ Stretch your arms out on the floor above your head; keep your neck straight by resting your forehead on the floor.
- ❖ As you lift a leg this time, also lift the opposite arm up, reaching out. Alternate sides.

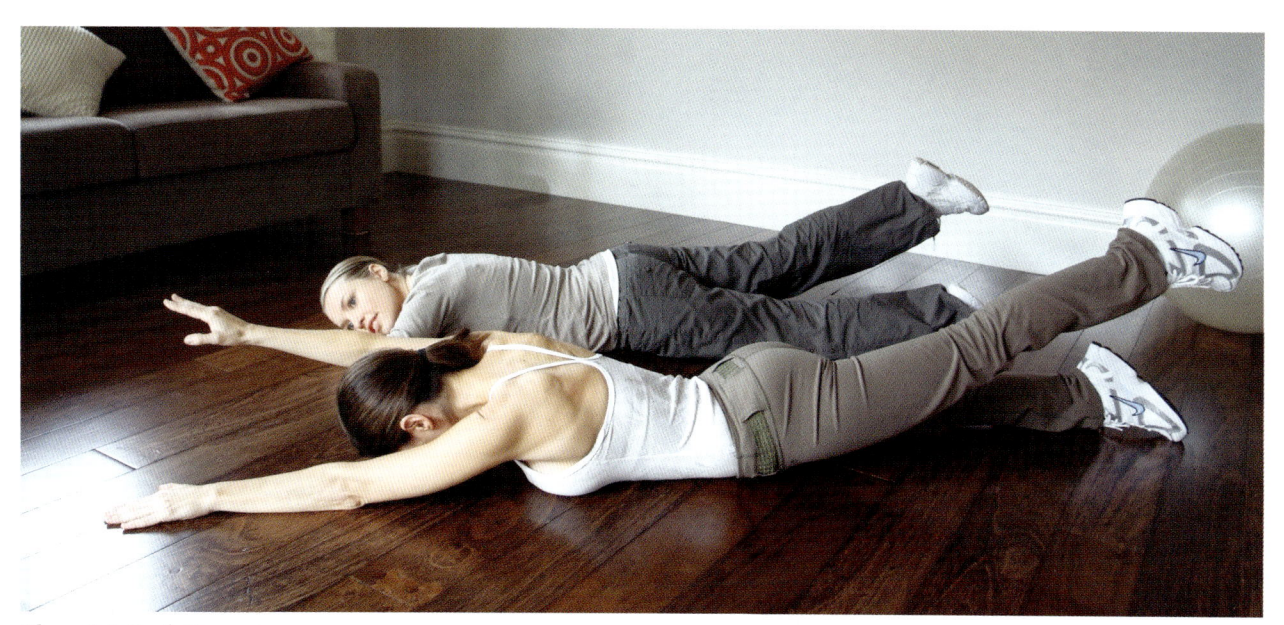

Photo 9.8 Back Extension

Stretching

Continue with the following stretches from the first six weeks:
- ❖ Arm crossover
- ❖ Neck stretch
- ❖ Seated toe touch
- ❖ Lower back stretch

And add the following two stretches to your routine.

CHEST OPENER (Photo 9.9)

This is a more advanced version of the stretch in the previous plan. Keep your back straight and tummy tight and you should feel the stretch across the front of your chest and shoulders.

- Take one end of a bath towel in each hand. Stretch your arms out wide in front of you. Slowly lift your arms up and over your head.
- Try to take your arms down to shoulder level, stretching the towel out behind you.

TRICEPS AND SHOULDER STRETCH (Photos 9.10)

The aim is to hold your hands behind your back. Don't forget to change sides.

- Holding a towel in one hand, take your arm up over your head and bend your elbow behind your head.
- Reach your other hand up your back to grab the towel. Walk your hands together along the towel and hold when you can't go any further. Aim to eventually drop the towel and clasp hands.

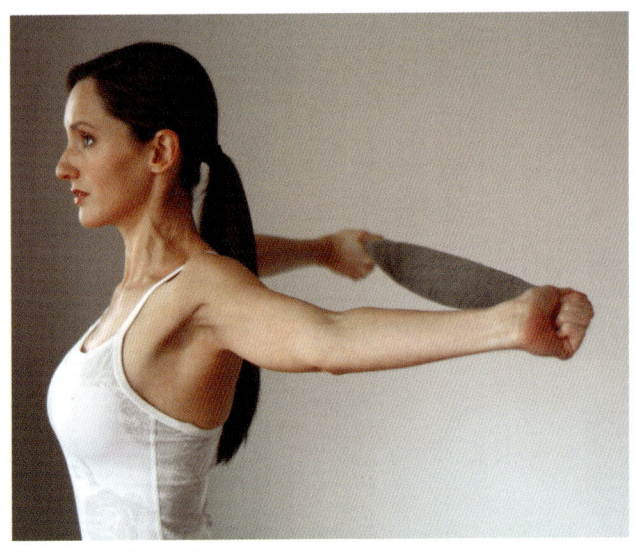

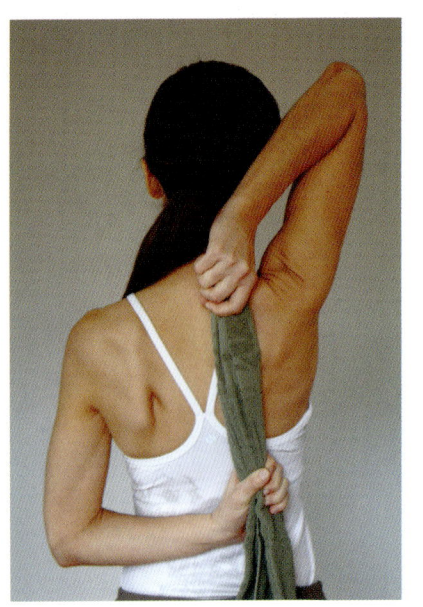

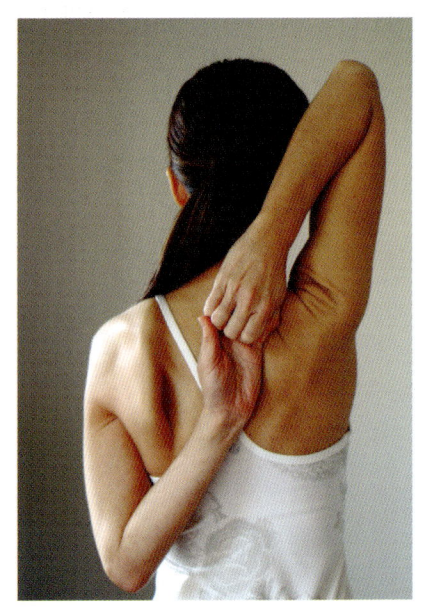

Photo 9.9 Chest Opener

Photos 9.10 Triceps and Shoulder Stretch

Scheduling

Aim to do the strength exercises three times a week. Schedule 20–30 minutes to do all the strength and flexibility exercises together, or keep doing your stretches after putting baby to bed (once a day is ideal) and do the strength work separately.

PLAN B

It happens to all of us. For days and weeks when you can't do it all, prioritise your exercise as follows.

- **First priority:** Pelvic floor and transverse abdominal exercises. Unless you are prohibited from doing so, do these every day, several times a day. You have to feed the baby, so do them then.
- **Second priority:** Walk, walk, walk. Whenever, wherever you can. It strengthens muscles, gets you fitter and helps you lose excess baby weight. If you can't walk, find another form of aerobic exercise to do, like swimming, a rowing machine or an exercise video. Just find something to get the heart rate up and do it every day.
- **Third priority:** Stretch. Hopefully you'll end up doing the stretches compulsively when you feel tight muscles or after strength exercises, and won't need separate time allocated to this. Until then, make an effort to stretch, as new mums can suffer lots of nasty aches and pains.
- **Fourth priority:** Strength. This is as important as the other forms of exercise, but at this point, don't pass on the walking for anything.

Don't forget to stay committed to proper nutrition. You have extra energy requirements if you're breastfeeding, so you'll probably feel hungry. Make smart choices and plan ahead so you don't undo your hard work or even put on more weight, which is not uncommon.

If you're breastfeeding but not losing weight, trim the fat from your meals but don't reduce the portion size, and *move more*. Remember: positive eating, five small meals, eat before you're starving and no skipping meals. Add the exercise and keep with it.

Action

Start squeezing—pelvic floors don't always mend themselves well

Pull your tummy in, any time you think of it, if that's where you want it to end up

Get your pram and walking shoes and go—now, today, no excuses!

Try the strength and stretching exercises and check your form in a mirror

If you miss a workout, do it tomorrow or do part of it—it doesn't have to be perfect . . . just give it a go!

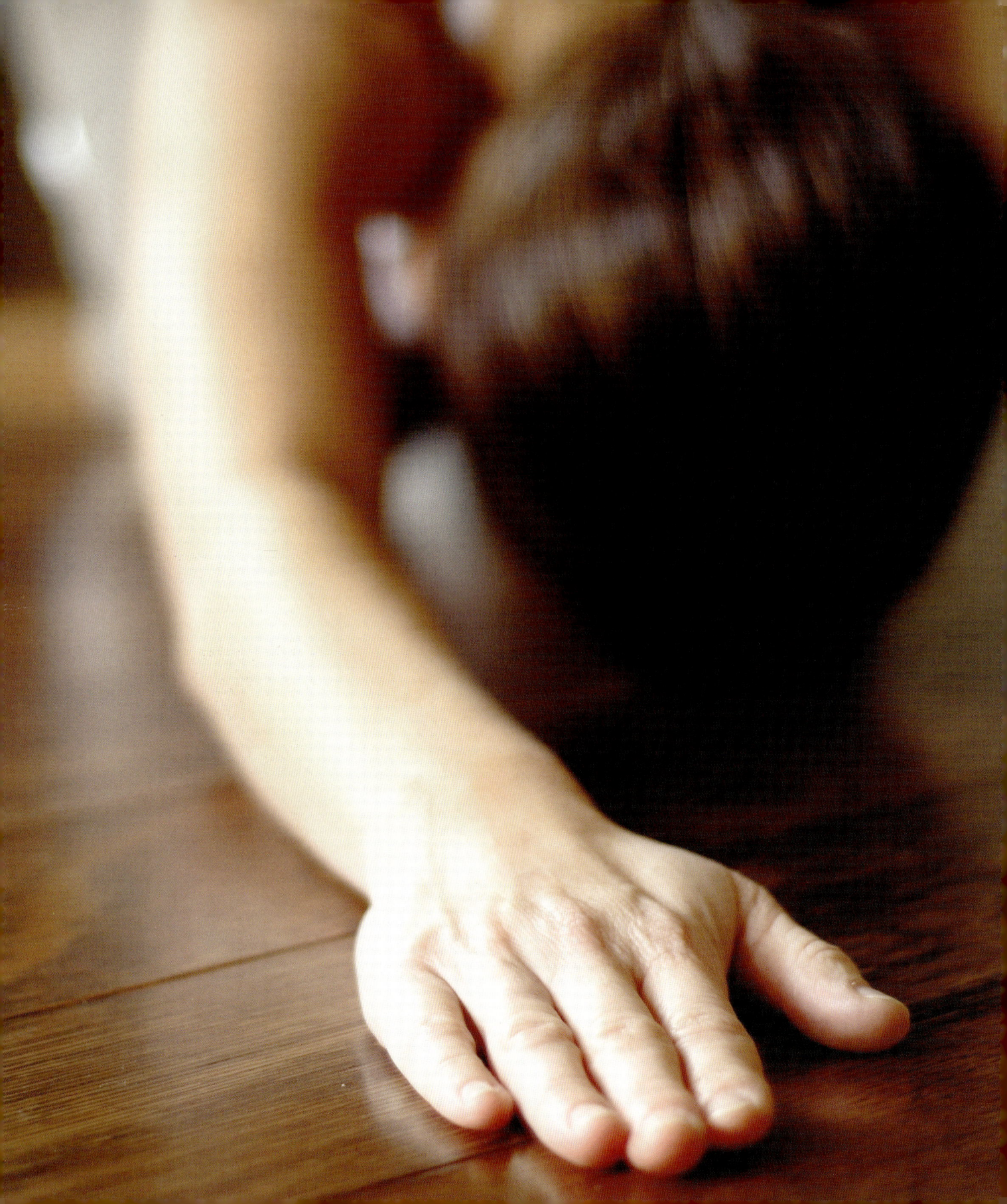

The second trimester after birth

By this stage your schedule has some degree of predictability. Stay committed by allocating a specific timeslot for a regular class, a game of social sport (like tennis) or a walk with a friend. A dog is a great friend to walk with—they know when it's time every day, they remind you energetically, keep begging until you go and are so grateful for your commitment. Walking with friends gives you an opportunity for adult conversation and also helps you stick to the program. Find other mums who are keen to exercise—you could all have a lot of fun at a social game or sports club. You can rotate to watch the babies and all get a workout.

Keep walking, and if you haven't added extra distance, speed or hills, now's the time. Aim to walk at least 30 minutes each day, or if it suits better, three or four longer walks per week. Involve baby in your walking program as she'll enjoy visiting a leafy park, busy shops or quiet beach. At home, put on music and do your strength and stretch exercises as she watches from a rocker. She'll love the stimulation: music and a show!

YOUR EXERCISE PLAN

Remember to monitor your progress using the exercise tracker (see Table 10.1). Keep walking as often as possible and doing pelvic floor and transverse abdominal exercises every day. If you're having trouble with the pelvic floor exercises and the muscles do not seem to be getting stronger and providing support when needed, this is a good time to check back with your obstetrician or gynecologist. For all the other exercises, do the prescribed number of sets and repetitions at least twice a day.

Ready?

What to do 12–24 weeks after the birth

Revised exercise trackers

Exercises to add as you get fitter

Reinvent previous exercises for new challenges

Notes on progression

Plan B, of course!

TABLE 10.1 Exercise tracker for second trimester after birth

EXERCISE/ AIM	SETS	REPS	MONDAY	TUESDAY	WEDNESDAY	THURSDAY	FRIDAY	SATURDAY	SUNDAY
Walk / 30 mins									
Pelvic floor/ slow and fast	6	10 each							
Transverse abs/plank	6	10							
Push-up	3	10							
Lunge	3 each side	10							
Back extension	3	10							
Crunch	2	10							
Oblique crunch	2 each side	10							
Triceps dip	3	10							
Chest opener stretch		3							
Arm crossover		3							
Triceps & shoulder stretch		3							
Neck stretch		3							
Seated toe touch		3							
Crossover back stretch		3							

Stamina

Thirty minutes of cardiovascular exercise per day, or three or four longer sessions per week. Make sure you work hard enough to get the heart rate up. You're at the point where you should be able to start making serious gains in your level of fitness. This will help you feel more energetic and tap into energy stores on the body, that is, spare baby weight. But don't forget to always listen to your body and if you need rest, take it.

Strength

Keep doing the exercises for the pelvic floor (remember, this one is for life!) and the transverse abdominal. If feeding sessions are less frequent or shorter, do these exercises several times a day while watching television, driving, preparing meals, washing up, folding laundry or doing other menial tasks. It's one way to get better value out of performing chores!

For all other exercises listed, start with as many repetitions and sets as you can do with good form and work up to the recommendations in the exercise tracker.

PUSH-UPS

Continue progressing through the levels from the last chapter.

If you're doing princess push-ups (on the knees), work on perfecting your form—keeping the transverse abdominals tight, back flat, hips down. Breathe and do them slowly.

If princess push-ups are too easy, you're either performing them too quickly or you're strong and should be doing them on your feet (see chapter 11).

THE 'PLANK'

If you're doing the transverse abdominal exercises well on your hands and knees, progress to these.

LEVEL 1 (Photo 10.1)

Start in the princess push-up position, but on your elbows instead of your hands. Keep your back straight, bottom down and pull your abs in—your body should be as straight as a plank. Hold this position as long as you can with good form, then rest and try again.

LEVEL 2 (Photo 10.2)

This is an advanced exercise and hard on your back if you don't have adequate abdominal support, so work up to this level.

Stay on your elbows, but balance on your toes instead of your knees, and keep the whole body straight. Hold this position as long as you can with good form, then rest and try again.

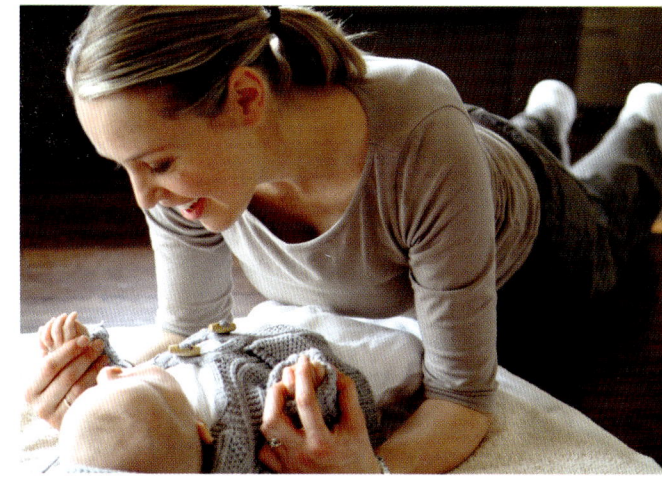

Photo 10.1 Level 1 Plank

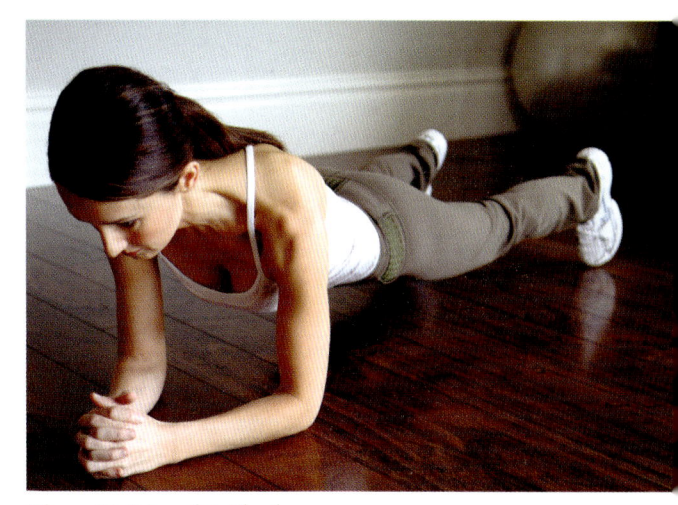

Photo 10.2 Level 2 Plank

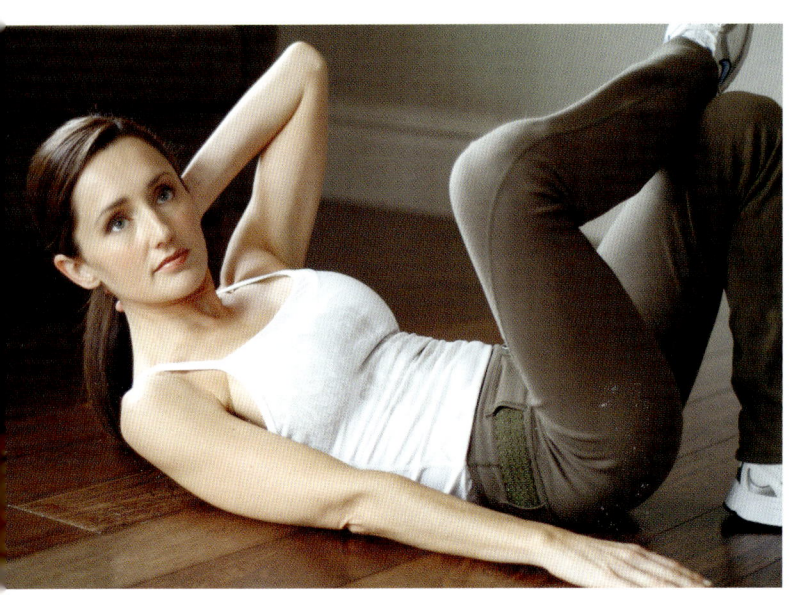

Photo 10.3 Oblique Crunch

OBLIQUE CRUNCH (Photo 10.3)

Once you have progressed through the abdominal crunches from the previous chapter, you're ready to add some variations for the obliques. These are also located on the front of the torso and run diagonally in 'V' and inverted 'V' patterns.

These should not be performed until abdominal separation has suitably healed.

Start in the crunch position. Cross your left leg over the right, knee turned out to the side. Place your right hand behind your neck for support.

Crunch diagonally across the torso. Think about taking your right shoulder towards your left knee by lifting your shoulders off the ground, then curling and twisting through the torso. Keep your elbow back and your neck straight and resist the urge to pull your head with your hand. Keep it slow and controlled.

Breathing technique: exhale as you lift, inhale going down. Work up to the sets and reps in the exercise tracker and don't forget to work both sides.

LUNGES (Photo 10.4)

When you've mastered the squats from the previous exercise program, try these. When done properly, lunges are one of the best 'compound' (using many muscles) exercises for the lower body.

As you get stronger, you can strap baby on in a sturdy pouch while doing squats or lunges. Keep good form, a wide stance for balance and have a chair back within reach as a safety precaution. As baby grows, you'll get progressively stronger and you'll both enjoy it.

Stand with your feet shoulder-width apart. Step one foot directly back into a wide lunge position. Your back foot should be up on the ball of the foot, with your toes pointing forward. Your feet should not be one in front of the other—keep them shoulder-width apart for stability.

Position your body in between your feet, and drop slowly straight down towards the ground. Bend the front knee to no more than a 90-degree angle. Keep your front knee in line with your front foot; the knee should not move forward over the front of the toes. This is not a forward lunging motion, it is a down-and-up motion. It's like being a pony on a carousel,

Photo 10.4 Lunges

going straight down and up on a pole. As you push up in the lunge, take your weight into the heel of the front foot and this will allow you to use the powerful muscles in the buttocks (gluteal mucles).

Count four seconds going down, and four seconds going up.

Do these slowly with good form and use a chair or wall if you need stabilising. Be conscious of keeping your pelvic floor and transverse abdominal tight.

Breathing: inhale going down, exhale pushing up. Try for 10 repetitions then change sides and work up to the recommendation in the tracker.

BACK EXTENSION

Your back and biceps (the muscles down the front of your upper arms) get progressive strength training as your baby gains weight. Every time you lift and carry baby your muscles are working hard!

Move to Level 2 of the back extension exercise from chapter 9 if you haven't already (see Photo 9.8). Concentrate on good form—exhaling as you lift the limbs, getting a good squeeze at the top of the movement, and controlling as you go down.

TRICEPS DIP

This exercise works the muscles at the back of the upper arm and some muscles in the shoulders. As always, perform this exercise slowly and with control.

LEVEL 1

Sit on the ground with your knees bent and your feet on the floor. Put your hands on the floor about 20–30 cm behind you, with your fingers pointing forwards towards your body.

With a straight back, lean backwards and take some weight on your hands. To perform the dip, bend your elbows and drop your body back towards the ground. Your elbows should point directly behind you.

Now push up through your hands to straighten your elbows. Be careful not to over-extend or 'lock' the elbow joint when straightening; keep it slightly bent so it feels like the muscles are working the whole time.

Breathing technique: inhale going down, exhale pushing back up. This level is usually easy, so move on as soon as you're ready.

LEVEL 2 (Photo 10.5)

Sit on the edge of a step, bench or sturdy chair, with your feet on the floor. Place your hands about shoulder-width apart on the front edge, with your fingers off the front edge pointing towards the ground.

Take your body weight onto the heel of your hand and walk your feet forward a couple of steps. Dip down by bending at the elbows until they are at a maximum 90-degree bend, then push back up again.

Stretching

Continue with the following stretches from chapter 9:
- Arm crossover
- Neck stretch
- Seated toe touch
- Chest opener
- Triceps and shoulder stretch

And add the following new stretch.

CROSSOVER BACK STRETCH (Photo 10.6)

You should feel this stretch mostly through the back and the buttocks (gluteal muscles). You may also feel it through the chest and the front of the shoulders.

Lie on the floor, on your back, with your knees up and feet on the floor. Gently drop your knees towards the floor to one side of the body. Take your arms straight out to the sides in line with your shoulders and try to keep both shoulder blades on the floor.

Roll your head to the opposite side to your legs. Relax and breathe into the stretch, then switch sides.

To stretch your biceps while lying there, stick out your thumbs and rotate your arms to give a 'thumbs-down' gesture.

To increase this stretch, pull your knees in closer to your chest and use the hand on the same side as your legs to push your legs down towards the ground.

Change sides by first contracting the transverse abdominal, then roll your knees and head slowly to the opposite side.

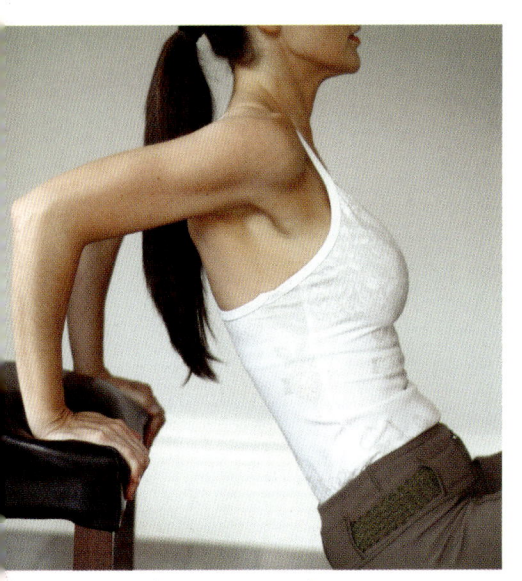

Photo 10.5 Level 2 Triceps Dip

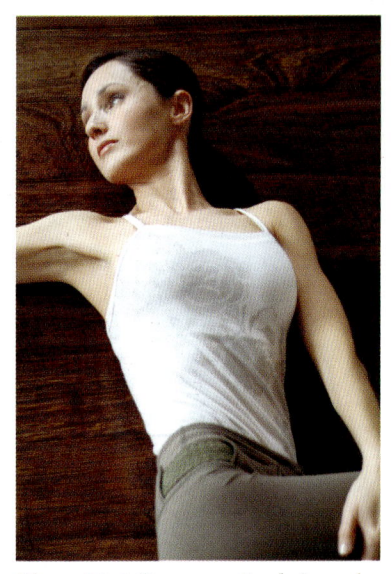

Photo 10.6 Crossover Back Stretch

Progression

I have only put in one exercise program for this three-month period, as there are enough levels and variations to keep you challenged for 12 weeks, particularly if you increase the intensity of your walking or add another activity. If you do the strength exercises two to three times every week they get easier. When the number of sets and repetitions are quite easy, progress to the harder options and work back up to the prescribed number.

Only ever do as many exercises as you can do with good form for effectiveness and safety. It's much better to do seven good slow lunges than 15 fast ones incorrectly.

Six months after giving birth, your joints should be stable enough to safely challenge yourself more. Aim to increase your range of motion by working further into the stretches. Remember, tension is all right, pain is not.

Scheduling

Keep referring to the exercise trackers at this stage as they are designed to help you establish habits and see how often you're actually fitting in the exercise. Have at least one exercise session per week locked in and build on this during the week. Schedule in some 'catch up' sessions on the weekend.

I have recommended doing the whole program at least twice a week. Remember, you can spread them throughout the day. It's surprising how often you can squeeze in a quick exercise or two.

PLAN B

If you have lost little or no weight or have gained weight six months after your baby was born, have a good hard think about what you've really been doing and eating. The golden rule is simply to move more and eat less.

If you find yourself here, look outside for support. Involve your partner, family or friends in your mission. Hopefully you'll find someone who will encourage you, help you—and even better, do it with you.

Action

Try to stay with the recommended progression—you'll have to be consistent, so keep it up

Revise your weekly planner each month—baby's feeding and sleeping schedule changes a lot during this period

If you've missed several weeks of exercise, consider changing activities to refresh your outlook

Find a friend to get in shape with you—it's more fun and adds extra motivation right when you may need it

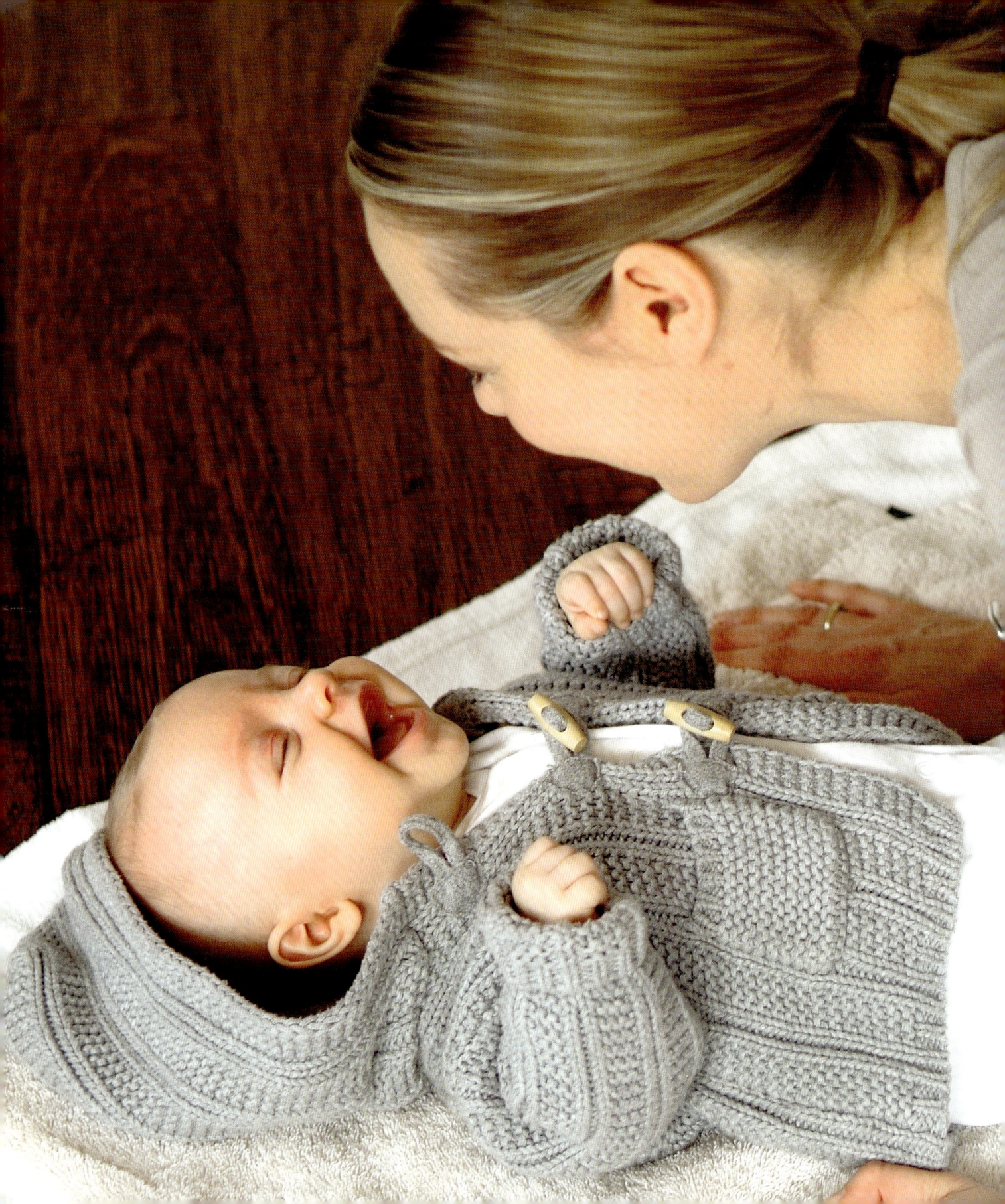

The third trimester after birth

There will have inevitably been ups and downs in all aspects of your life since the birth. Now that your baby is six months old it's a good time to evaluate the net effect of your new lifestyle. Unless you've had complications, nine months is a reasonable time to get most things back into shape after a baby; you've now got three months to go.

Some body parts take longer to get back to where they were, and others will always be different. Stay realistic about your schedule, your lifestyle and what you expect to achieve. If you're disappointed with how you've done so far, consider what you could do differently. Have you prioritised your health? You have to be willing to do what it takes to get what you want.

Also remind yourself that 'perfect' has no place in health goals . . . fit, fabulous and full of energy is what you want.

If you've stuck with the program, you should be reasonably fit and strong and losing some excess baby baggage. However, some women lose weight relatively easily in the first few months after a baby and then reach a plateau where they stop. If this happens, don't panic! You don't have to carry the last five kilos for the rest of your life—you simply need to make some changes. Don't worry, this is not about training more, just training smarter. If you've stopped losing weight, your body has temporarily found an equilibrium where energy in = energy out. You need to find new ways to tip the scales once more in your favour.

If you keep performing the same activity over time, your body gets more efficient and it becomes easier to do. In other words, you get fitter, which is great. But to keep moving forward, you need to increase the

Ready?

Ways to jump-start if you've stalled

A new exercise tracker

Modifications to make your workout even more challenging

Keeping it super simple, super fast but super effective

Scheduling ideas

The countdown to your nine-month goals

difficulty and challenge your body again. For example, do you recall how hard you were breathing on your first walk up a decent hill with the pram? Then how it became easier the more you did it? Your cardiovascular system and every muscle involved with this activity became accustomed to the demands of your walk. If you went swimming now, even if you're reasonably fit, it might be quite a hard workout if you haven't been training the body in this way. This comes back to the principle of cross training.

Basically, if you no longer get your heart rate up or use enough energy walking, it's time to try jogging, interval sprints, swimming, dancing, cycling, rowing, or another way to challenge your body. If all else fails, just walk faster, further, or up bigger hills than you're used to.

And don't forget to check your eating habits. Make sure you're still getting plenty of water, fresh fruit and vegies, lean protein and complex carbs. Check that high-sugar and high-fat junk foods haven't crept in on a regular basis—remember, it all adds up!

Reviewing and remodelling your program at regular intervals helps with motivation and keeps you moving towards your fitness goals. So get out your schedule and put in the programs for the next three months.

The exercise tracker in this chapter is different. During the last six months my advice was to do as much exercise as you could and to track your progress. If you've made the effort and been reasonably consistent, you should be used to exercising. Now you can aim to complete two full-body workouts a week, marking each exercise under the weekly column.

Again there is only one program, with exercise modifications to keep it challenging but short. There are certainly many other exercises you could add, but this program gives a fast, all-round workout without obsessing over isolating specific muscles. The exercise program does not contain the stretches this time as you should be used to doing them regularly by now. Just continue these as previously—after cardiovascular exercise, while relaxing or after the strength exercises.

Progression through the different exercise variations is very individual. I have scheduled them with an 'average' progression in mind, if you manage the recommended amount of exercise. But all of this depends on specific factors such as how often you exercise, how strong you were when you started, previous training, your body type, how your body responds and your natural strengths. Some women may still be doing Level 1 push-ups at six months, others may be doing them on their toes after six weeks.

Move at your own speed, but keep challenging your body. If an exercise becomes too easy, take the recommended steps to increase the difficulty. If you have the time and facilities to train more or harder—fantastic, go for it! Chapter 12 outlines some exercise options using basic home equipment.

YOUR EXERCISE PLAN

Here is your new exercise tracker for you to monitor your progress every week. Do each exercise twice a week and record sets and repetitions as follows; 12/12/10, or if you do two sets, 10/8, for example. For abdominals, do two sets of straight crunches and two sets of oblique crunches (from chapter 10).

TABLE 11.1 Exercise tracker for third trimester after birth

BODY PART	EXERCISES	SETS	REPS	WEEK 1	WEEK 2	WEEK 3	WEEK 4	WEEK 5	WEEK 6
LEGS	Squats	3	10						
	Lunges	3 each side	10						
ARMS	Dips	3	12						
CHEST	Push-ups	3	12						
BACK	Extensions	3	10						
ABS	Crunches	4	10						

Stamina

Do at least 30 minutes each day of cardiovascular exercise, or three or four longer sessions a week.

Increase your level of incidental exercise, such as walking to the shops, dancing, kicking a ball with preschoolers or even vacuuming!

Strength

- Continue your pelvic floor exercises.
- Transverse abdominal exercises: continue to progress through the levels described in chapter 10.
- Aim to do all the other strength exercises twice a week. That means ticking off each box on the tracker twice each week.

LEGS

Mix it up with the lunges and squats. Try the following variations and change them on your exercise program every few weeks for interest as well as good all-round leg training.

Make squats and lunges harder by adding weight: hold bags of rice, buckets of sand, two litre plastic milk bottles (with handles) filled with water, or preferably a set of hand weights. When lunging, hold a weight beside your body in each hand. When squatting, hug a weight close to your chest with both arms.

DYNAMIC LUNGES (Photo 11.1)

These can be done on level ground or on a step.
- Stand with your feet together. Take a big step forward, far enough so that the front knee drops down over your ankle, not over the front of your foot.
- Drop into a lunge, then push back up and step your feet back together into the starting position. Alternate legs.

TRAVELLING LUNGES

These are done taking giant steps and travelling forwards.
- Take a big step forward and drop down into a lunge, then push up and step your other foot forward into a lunge. You should travel forward in a straight line.
- Watch that the front knee doesn't bend more than 90 degrees or project beyond the front foot when you lunge.

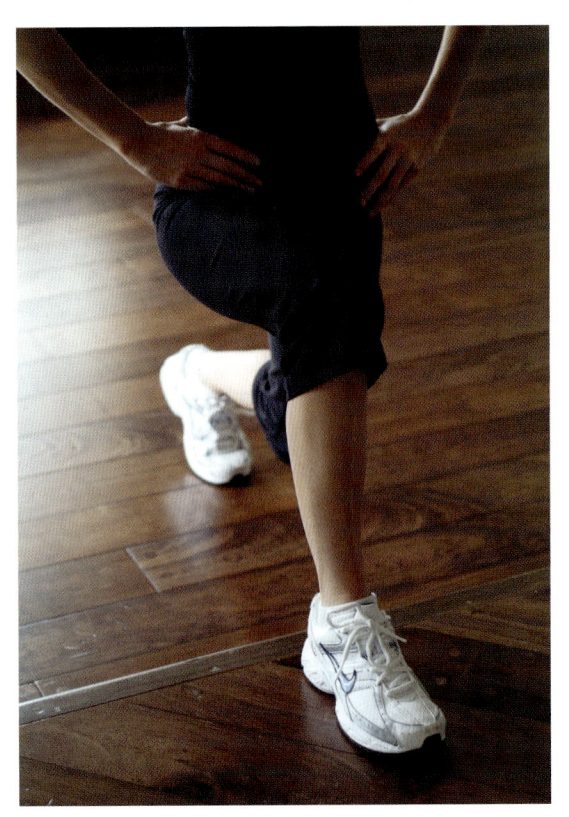

Photo 11.1 Dynamic Lunge

SQUATS
- Try squats with a narrow, ski-like stance. (See Photo 11.2)
- Try squats with a wide stance, with your feet turned out. Keep your body upright and 'sit' down. (See Photo 11.3)

TRICEPS AND SHOULDERS
Continue with your tricep dips and progress to Level 2 as described in chapter 10. (See Photo 10.5)

PUSH-UPS ON THE TOES (Photo 11.4)
If princess push-ups are too easy, you can progress to push-ups on the toes and really impress your partner (or put him to shame!). Push-ups on the toes require a lot of upper body strength, and are particularly challenging for women as we generally have narrower shoulders than men compared to the rest of our bodies. Focus on good form and breathing at all times.

Start in the princess push-up position and straighten your legs to take the weight onto your toes. Aim for a straight line from your toes through your knees and hips to your shoulders—no bottom sticking up or saggy tummy.

Keep the transverse abdominal contracted and perform the push-up exercise as usual.

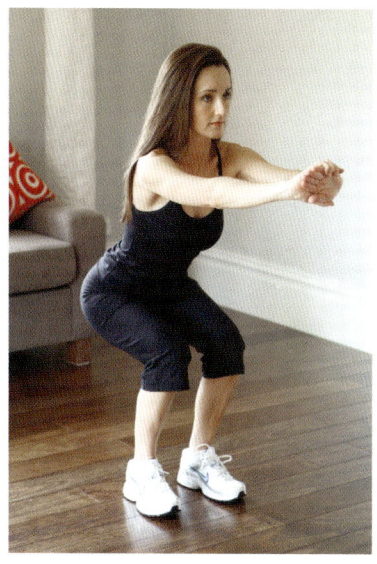

Photo 11.2 Narrow Squat

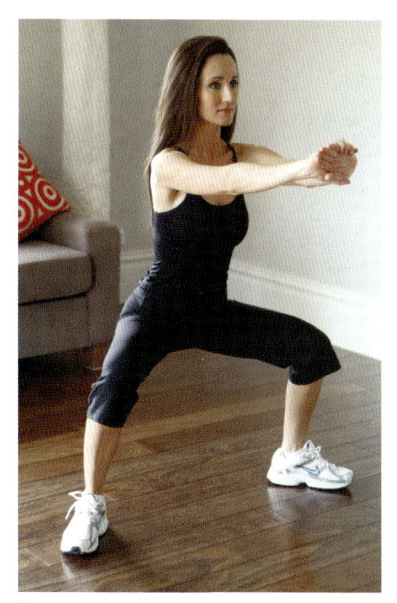

Photo 11.3 Wide Squat

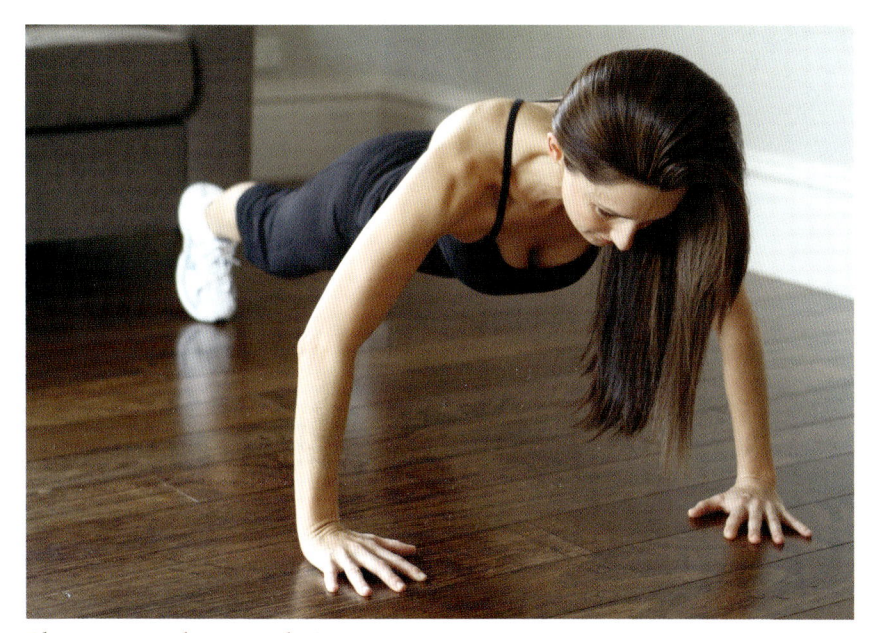

Photo 11.4 Push-ups on the Toes

BACK

Keep doing the back extension exercises. Don't forget the back stretches—after the exercise when your muscles are warm.

Whenever lifting baby remember to switch on your transverse abdominal to protect your back. For muscle balance, also try to switch the side you carry baby on. Your biceps and upper back get progressive strength training every time you pick baby up and this is why I haven't specifically targeted these areas with other exercises.

ABDOMINALS

A combination of straight and oblique crunches will keep this area strong, but remember you don't need thousands of these. Good-quality crunches which are slow and controlled keep the torso functionally strong and give nice contours (provided they're not hiding behind several inches of padding).

If you have an exercise ball, you can progress to doing your abdominal work on this now. Chapter 12 gives details for this option.

Stretching

Continue doing the following stretches from previous chapters regularly:
- Neck stretch
- Arm crossover
- Seated toe touch
- Chest opener
- Triceps and shoulder stretch
- Crossover back stretch

Scheduling

Once again, it's up to you whether you do all exercises together, or split the routine up and spread it throughout the day or week. I recommend you schedule in specific times to do it and not count on 'getting around to it' when you're not busy—it only gets busier as baby spends less time asleep and you have more outings, play dates and activities.

An easy scheduling idea is to split the six strength exercises in this program into three groups of two exercises (see Table 11.1) and do it six days a week (each group twice). It's not as much commitment as it seems;

about 10 minutes a day, easily done when you get out of bed or before you have a shower or while dinner's cooking.

PLAN B

If you are struggling with exercising, review your schedule, then focus on the area of fitness you need most. If you need to lose weight, devote as much time as you can to walking or cardiovascular exercise. Although the strength training builds energy-burning muscle, give yourself a headstart with a few weeks of harder, longer cardio work. Once that's going well, add the resistance training back in.

Daily life with an infant can be so engrossing that it's hard to look at the big picture. If you're not seeing the physical results you'd like, it's easy to become discouraged and think 'why bother'. But focus on how far you've come since the birth, what you were like before and how you would like to be in the not-too-distant future.

All the little daily efforts add up to the body and the health profile you earn. And this remains true for the rest of your life, babies or not.

WHEN YOUR NINE MONTHS ARE UP

I mentioned previously that as it takes nine months for your body to prepare for a baby, it is reasonable to take nine months to get your body back after having a baby.

Of course, there are many reasons why women don't reach all their fitness, health or body goals in this time period. But if this is the case for you, it's important to determine whether these reasons are truly something outside your control, like ongoing medical complications for you or baby, or whether they are just excuses.

If you're giving yourself as much as a year to get back in shape, really make it a deadline and commit. A year is generous in terms of recovering from pregnancy. You can make huge lifestyle changes in 12 months which dramatically affect your health. Use the same programs for the first nine months, but use each program for longer, until you're ready to move on. Then check out the next chapter for further fitness gains with basic home equipment. You can take your fitness to the next level—that is, even fitter than before baby!

Action

If you're slipping in the nutrition stakes, do another food diary and check it against the healthy eating criteria in chapter 5

Try a new activity to keep you challenged in body and mind

Don't forget to stretch— one day, put on relaxing music and stretch for an hour; it will feel like a mini holiday!

Don't stress over what you haven't done—just go for a walk, now

If you need more time to get in shape, take it, but use it well

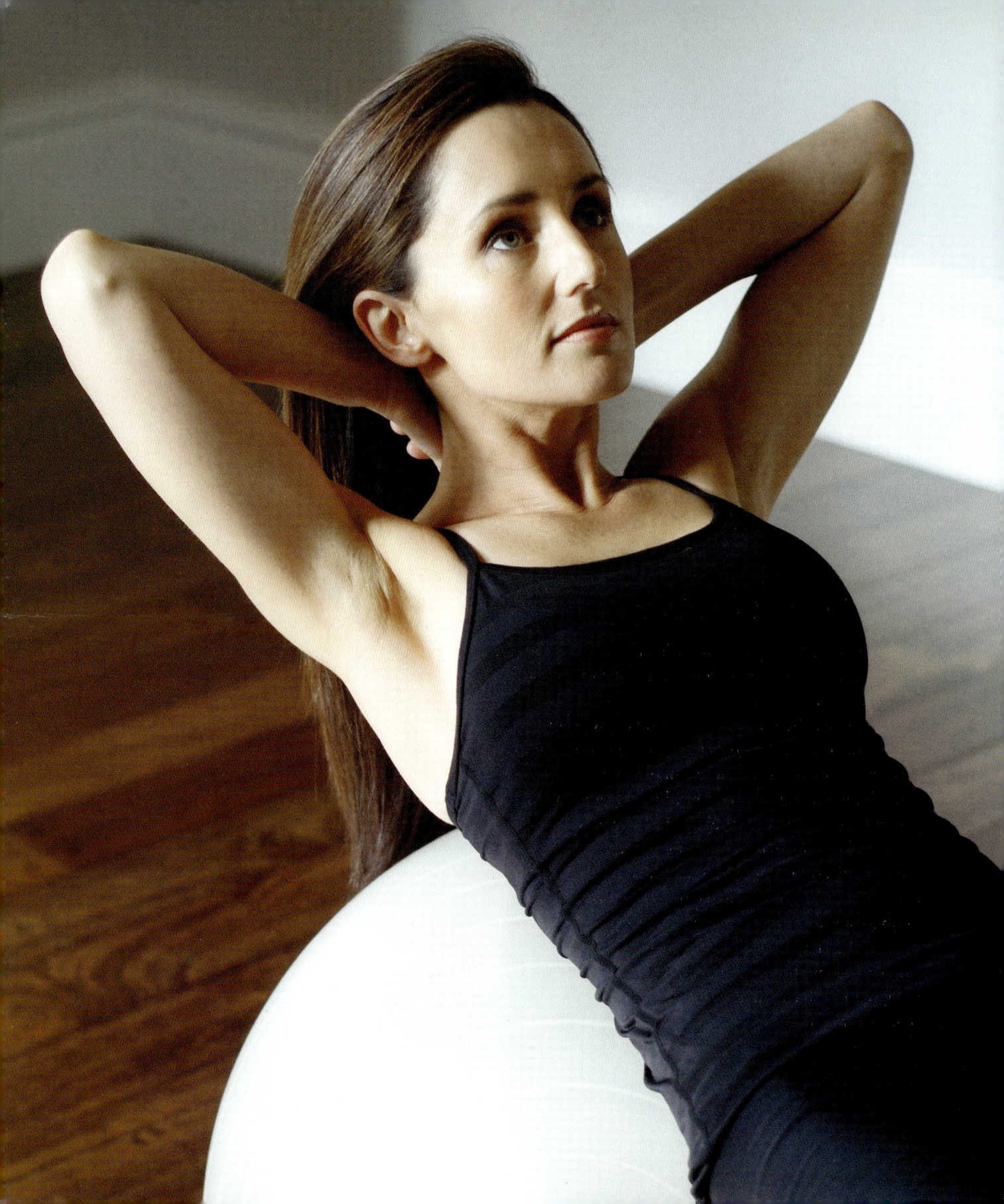

Beyond basics: Training with equipment

Ready?

Using equipment and getting help with future training

Two new programs that fit easily in a busy schedule

Exercise with weights— for women only!

Get on the ball for harder abdominal work

So far I have focussed on exercising without equipment as it's the easiest, most accessible option. It minimises obstacles and excuses to exercising and is perfectly effective. But I've also mentioned that resistance training is the secret weapon to getting into great shape for life, and using equipment significantly enhances this. The ongoing benefits in terms of bone density and body composition greatly improve your quality of life— not only now but for the rest of your life.

Lifting weights creates the shape and firmness many women want: defined shoulders to balance and complement the curves below, a strong shapely midsection, a firm backside and contoured legs. Most women are surprised by how resistance training changes their bodies!

This chapter covers exercising with basic equipment, challenging your body in new ways to push through plateaus in your training and inject variety. The exercises can be added or substituted into the previous programs at any stage you're ready, after the six-week check-up. If you've reached your post-baby fitness goals, training with equipment will take you to the next level and get you in the best shape ever, no matter what your age or how many babies you have!

See chapter 7 for details on the basic equipment used for exercises in this chapter. If you use free weights, make sure you can finish at least eight repetitions with good form for each exercise with the chosen weight. If you can't do this, choose a lighter weight, otherwise you risk injury. Work up to the recommended number of sets and repetitions as detailed in this chapter's exercise trackers (e.g. three sets of 10 reps). Keep with it, and when you can regularly do three sets of 15, move to a heavier weight.

A NOTE ON THE EXERCISES

There is an extensive range of exercise options when using equipment. I've chosen some standard, efficient exercises to get you started lifting weights. It really helps to do these in front of a mirror occasionally to check if you're moving correctly as shown in the photos.

If you master these exercises and want to progress to more advanced weight training, you'll find an infinite number of resources listing exercise options online. Better still, book an appointment with an exercise physiologist to tailor a program especially for you. Remember, Medicare rebates now apply for allied health professionals such as these, and many private health funds will also cover part of the cost.

If you have trouble with your form or progression, it's well worth consulting an exercise physiologist, exercise scientist or suitably qualified personal trainer every few months to keep you on track and renew your program. (When choosing a personal fitness trainer, as qualifications vary widely, look for recognised tertiary education in the field and professional registration and insurance.) It works out much cheaper than a gym membership, and they will make sure your program can be done at home, when you want, with the resources you have available.

The following exercises are designed using dumbbells, as they are simple and convenient in most situations. Feel free to substitute other types of weights, bands or machines, but seek professional advice on how to modify the exercises correctly.

YOUR EXERCISE PLAN

One tactic I use for women not keen on weight training is to perform only one exercise a day of the seven listed in the program (see Table 12.1). It only takes four or five minutes to do a few sets of one exercise plus a stretch for the appropriate body part. Using this one-a-day strategy proves how easy it is to slot a whole-body workout into the busiest week.

When you're successfully completing one exercise a day, string a few together for a slightly longer workout two or three times a week. The second program offers a two-day split to try as an alternative (see Table 12.2). Alternate Day 1 and Day 2, any day of the week, as often as you like. How quickly you change to heavier weights depends on how often you train and how your body responds. Record the number of sets and repetitions and also the weight of your dumbbells—starting light and progressing to heavier ones.

Don't forget about regular cardiovascular exercise to keep your energy and fitness levels up and perhaps trim the last of the baby weight.

TABLE 12.1 Exercise tracker: One-a-day program

DAY	BODY PART & EXERCISE		WEEK 1	WEEK 2	WEEK 3	WEEK 4	WEEK 5	WEEK 6
MONDAY	LEGS	Ball leg curl or Lunges						
TUESDAY	ARMS	Triceps extension						
WEDNESDAY		Bicep curl						
THURSDAY	SHOULDERS	Upright row						
FRIDAY	CHEST	Chest fly						
SATURDAY	BACK	Dumbbell row						
SUNDAY	ABS	Crunches						

TABLE 12.2 Exercise tracker: Two-day split program

DAY	BODY PART & EXERCISE		WEEK 1	WEEK 2	WEEK 3	WEEK 4	WEEK 5	WEEK 6
DAY 1	LEGS	Ball leg curl or Lunges						
	BACK	Dumbbell row						
	SHOULDERS	Upright row						
DAY 2	CHEST	Chest fly						
	ARMS	Triceps extension						
		Bicep curl						
	ABS	Crunches						

Legs

Lunges are such a great compound exercise, so add hand weights and keep them going. Alternate with squats as well.

LEG CURL

If you have a ball, this is a great exercise for your repertoire. It targets the hamstrings—the muscles along the back of the thighs—and also works many others. It requires decent core strength to stabilise, so work up through the levels, always keeping good form.

LEVEL 1 (Photo 12.1)

- Lie on the floor, facing up, with your arms resting beside your body. Bend your knees up and rest your heels on top of the ball.
- Roll the ball in until it touches the backs of your thighs and your feet are flat on the ball. This should be easy and just gets your form ready for the real exercise.

LEVEL 2 (Photo 12.2)

- Start in the same position as Level 1. Keep your arms on the floor beside your body for stability.
- Raise your hips off the floor so the hip joint is straight. Bend your knees and roll the ball in towards your backside, pulling your knees into your chest. Extend your legs again and lastly lower your hips to the floor. Do this slowly and with control. The movement sequence is: lift hips up, roll in, roll out, then lower hips.
- Remember to breathe: exhale on the hardest part, which is pulling the ball in.

LEVEL 3

This is advanced, so only attempt it once you have mastered Level 2. It is the same exercise, except the stability given by the arms is taken away.

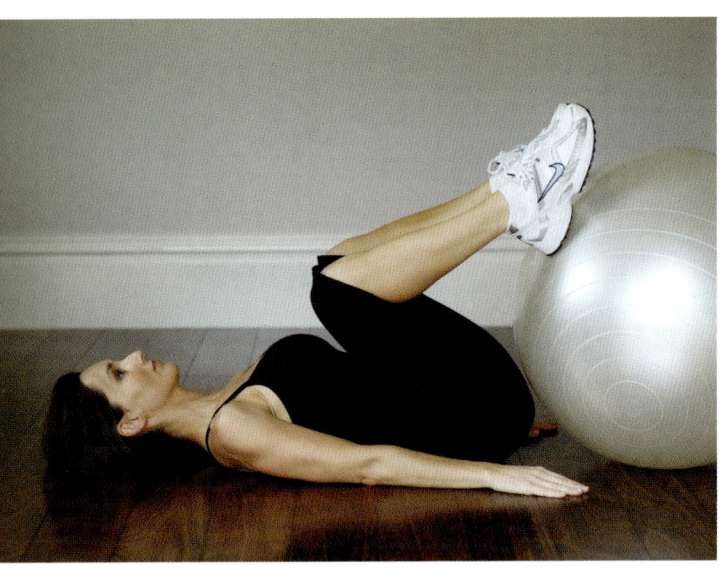

Photo 12.1 Level 1 Leg Curl

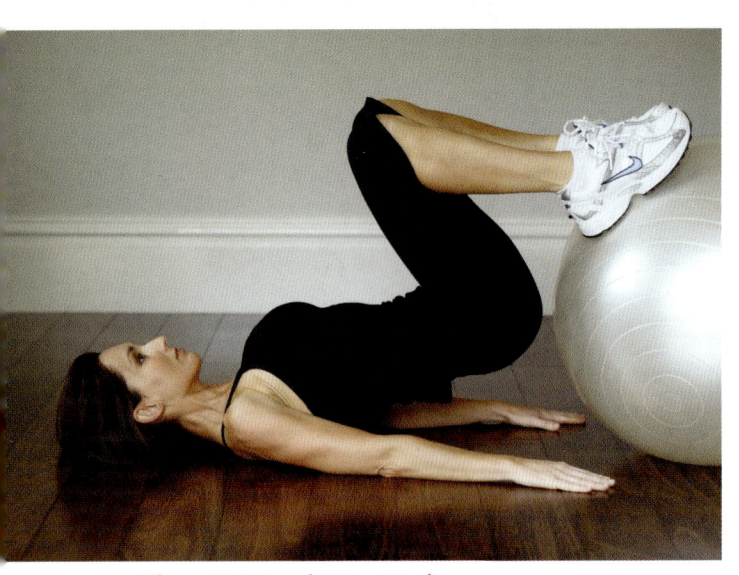

Photo 12.2 Level 2 Leg Curl

- Try the leg curl first with your elbows on the ground beside you, hands up in the air.
- When you're ready for the next stage, rest your arms above your head or on your chest throughout the exercise.

Arms

TRICEPS EXTENSION (Photo 12.3)

This exercise is safer on the neck and does not require as much flexibility as overhead triceps presses. Also, you get to lie down and take a break!

- Lie face up on the floor or bench, with your knees bent. Hold a dumbbell in each hand in a 'hammer' grip (wrists facing in towards each other).
- Press the weights straight up to the ceiling directly above your shoulders and hold; this is the starting position.
- Keeping your elbows where they are (above the shoulders), bend at the elbow joint to lower the weights down beside your head (watch out for the ears!), and then extend back up.
- Do this slowly and exhale as you lift.

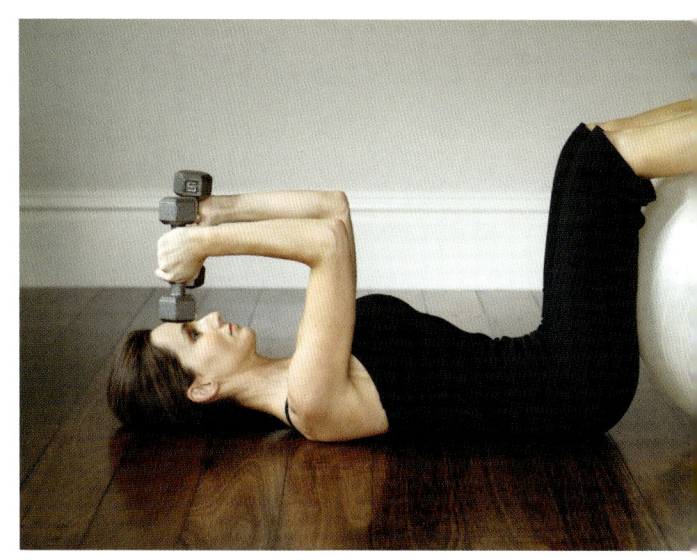

Photo 12.3 Triceps Extension

BICEP CURL (Photo 12.4)

This works the muscles on the front of the upper arm. Throughout this exercise it's important to keep your elbows right beside your waist, as though they are pinned there, and don't swing through the movement, as often seen in the 'big boys' room at the gym. It's cheating and dangerous. If you can't do this exercise under control it means the weight is too heavy.

- Start in a staggered stance—like a surfing stance: feet shoulder-width apart, with one foot further forward than the other, the knees soft and with equal weight between both feet.
- Take one dumbbell in each hand, hold them with your wrists facing forward as though you're holding a long barbell (or use a long barbell if you like).
- Keep your abs tight and exhale as you bend the elbows and lift the weights up towards the shoulders. Then lower slowly.

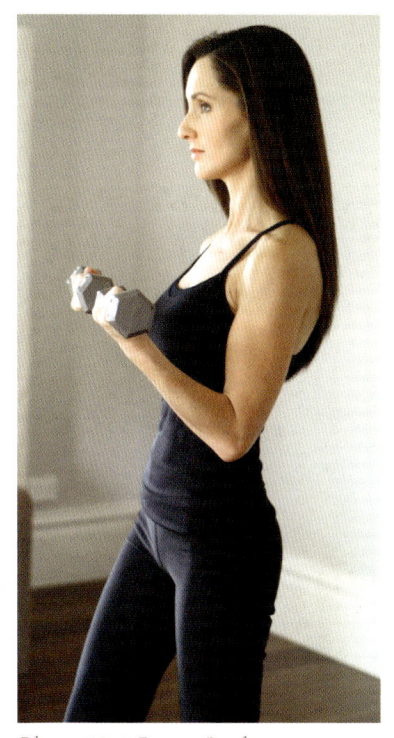

Photo 12.4 Bicep Curl

BEYOND BASICS: TRAINING WITH EQUIPMENT 193

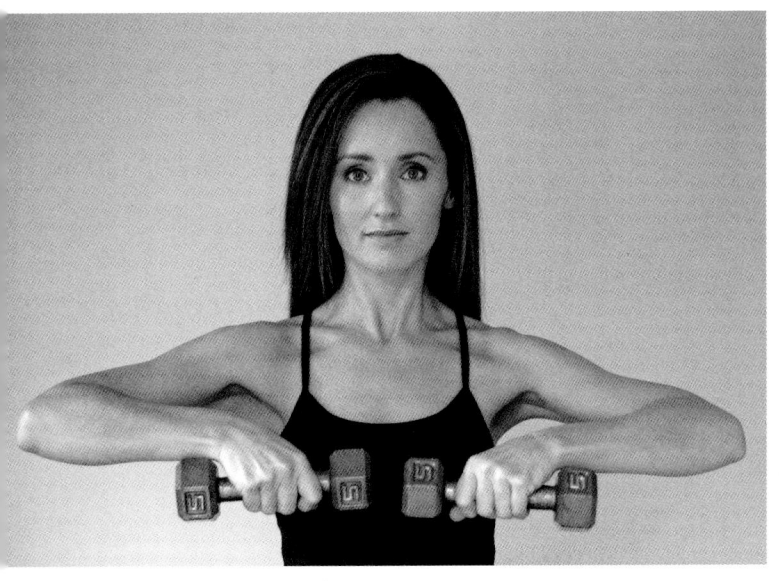

Photo 12.5 Upright Row

Shoulders

UPRIGHT ROW (Photo 12.5)

To get the right form for this one, imagine wearing rubber wading pants, grabbing the waistband and hitching them up really high to go fly fishing—that's how this exercise should look and feel.

- Stand in a staggered stance. Tighten your abs to stabilise. Use a dumbbell in each hand, or a long bar, with your hands about shoulder-width apart.
- Rotate your wrists forward so the back of your hands face out, so when you pull up your elbows stick out to the sides.
- As you exhale, raise the weights up to about nipple height—depending on how much they've sagged!—but keep your hands a few inches below the shoulders. Your elbows should point straight out to the sides, with the upper arm parallel to the floor. Keep your shoulders down (don't shrug). Slowly lower the weights and repeat.
- Go slowly—three or four seconds each way and exhale on the lift.

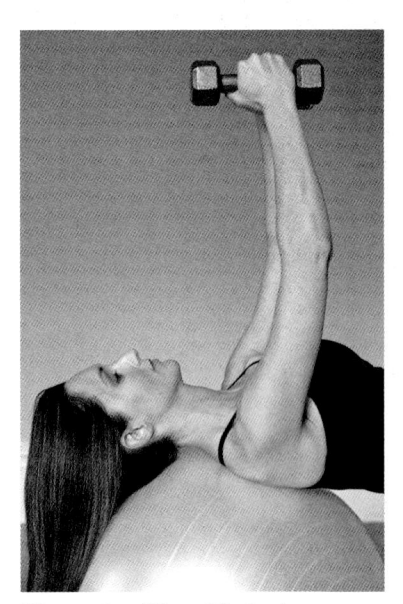

Photo 12.6 Chest Fly (up)

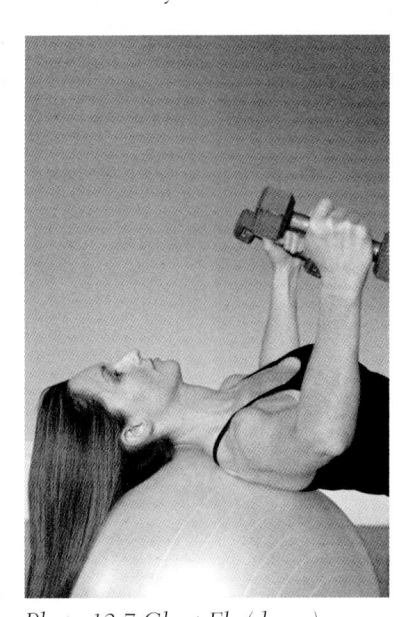

Photo 12.7 Chest Fly (down)

Chest

CHEST FLY (Photos 12.6 and 12.7)

The action in this exercise is like giving a big bear hug to a tree. It works the chest muscles in a slightly different way to push-ups.

- Lie on a ball in a slight incline position (with your head higher than your hips) or on a bench (flat or inclined). Tighten the abs for support especially if you're on a ball. If you're on a bench, bend your knees and place your feet flat on the bench or floor to reduce stress on the lower back.

- With a dumbbell in each hand, press your arms up straight above your chest. Turn your wrists to face each other. Start with the weights together and a slight bend in the elbow.
- Slowly take the weights out to the sides, stop when they are beside the shoulders (don't stretch the chest out too far), then exhale as you push back up and in, so the weights are together.

Back

DUMBBELL ROW (Photo 12.8)

This exercise works muscles on the upper back and the back of the shoulder.

- Place one knee and the same hand on a bench or chair. This is like being on your hands and knees on one side of your body, torso parallel to the ground. Keep the knee of the standing leg slightly bent and the abs tight.
- Take a dumbbell in your free hand in a 'hammer' grip (wrist in), with your arm straight and the weight hanging towards the ground.
- Exhale as you pull the weight straight up, the elbow bending behind you until the weight is next to your waist. Then slowly lower.
- Don't forget to change sides.

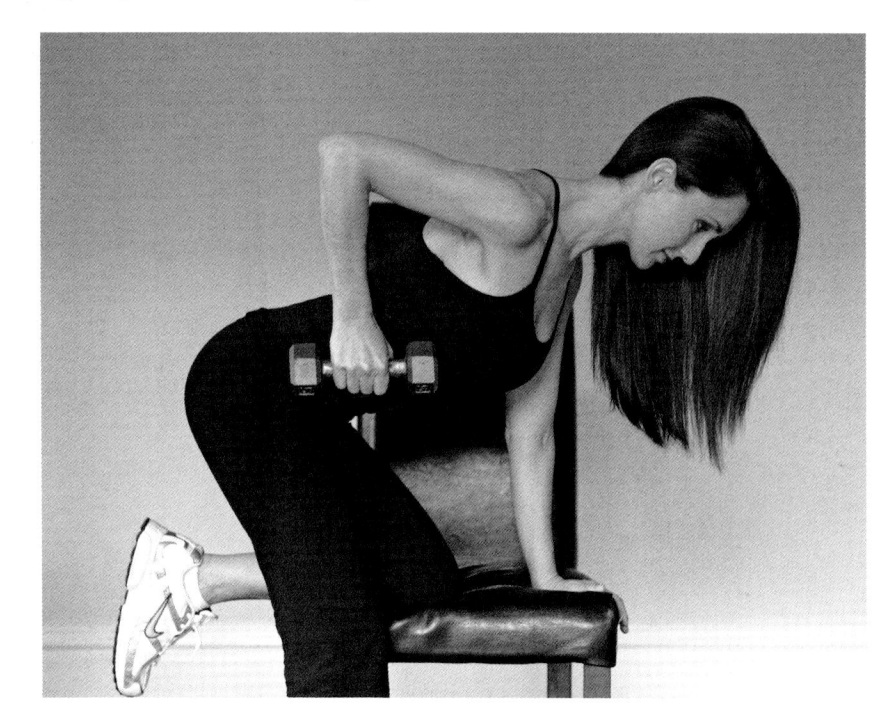

Photo 12.8 Dumbbell Row

Action

Gather some exercise equipment—remember you don't need to buy it brand new

Find a safe, convenient place to store it, away from little hands

Start the exercises slowly, and always prioritise good form over heavy weights

Consistency pays off—it won't happen overnight, but it will happen!

Abdominals

CRUNCHES ON THE BALL (Photo 12.9)

These are harder than they look if done properly. Make sure you have good transverse abdominal strength and stability before trying them. If you don't have a ball, continue with the abdominal variations from the previous chapters.

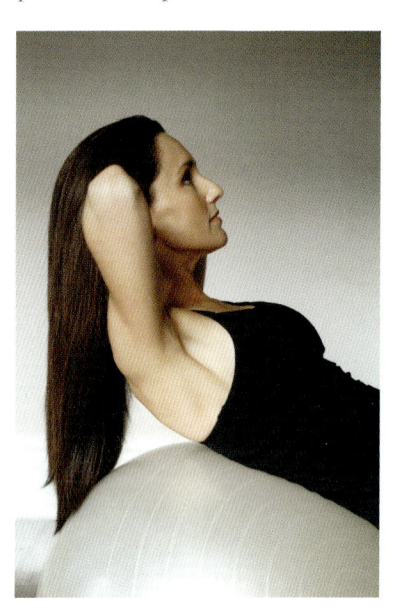

Photo 12.9 Crunches on Ball

- Sit on the ball, take a couple of steps forward and roll your back down the ball. Keep your feet about hip-width apart, and your tail bone and lower back in contact with the ball.
- Place your hands behind your head for support. Always keep your neck in line with your spine—never crunch or bend through the neck.
- Before crunching, contract your transverse abdominals to support your spine. Now perform crunches as you did on the floor, exhaling as you curl through the torso (not the neck), bringing your ribs towards your hips ... slowly and under control.
- To make it harder: step backwards and roll the tail bone higher on the ball. This gives less back support. Or try oblique crunches across the torso—cross one leg over the other, keeping one foot on the ground. Just keep it slow and breathe!

Stretching

Keep up the stretches from the previous chapters. When you lift weights you are repeatedly contracting—which means shortening and tightening—your muscles. It is important to continue flexibility training to prevent injury, maintain range of motion and prevent perpetually tight, aching muscles.

Try a yoga or flexibility class or DVD for all-over stretching and to add variety to your routine.

Keep up the good work!

If you're still working towards your goals after 12 months remember these words: **Never give in, never give in. Never, never, never ...** (Winston Churchill)

There are two easy ways to ensure you never get what you want; do not even start or just give up. And the only way to get it is to stay focussed and choose to do what it takes every day to move one step closer.

If you've more or less reached your fitness goals, well done—you should be proud! Now it's just a matter of maintaining what you've achieved and your healthy lifestyle and habits.

If you've finished having babies, then you have your body back to yourself and it's reassuring to know that the results of your hard work will stay with you.

If you're planning to have another baby, keep in mind that all the work you do (or don't do) has a cumulative effect on how healthy you are during and after your next pregnancy. Being in shape before you're pregnant means you aren't starting from scratch afterwards, or carrying compounding luggage from one pregnancy to the next. And that can only be a good thing!

This book is only a starting point for what I hope will become for you a way of life, a commitment, an area of further exploration—if it hasn't already—or, at the very least, a hobby. As you raise your babies, know that your commitment to a healthy lifestyle will give your family many gifts which are well worth the effort: good nutrition and exercise habits to last a lifetime, protection against certain lifestyle diseases, self-esteem and, above all, a fit mother ready for the challenge.

Index

abdominal exercises 157–59
  transverse 158–59
alcohol 61–63

baby blues 27
body composition 49–52, 54
body mass index (BMI) 50

carbohydrate 57–60
  recommended intake 69
cross-training 127–28

energy, definition 47
environment 14–15
exercise
  during pregnancy 137–51
  first trimester after birth 153–71
  planning 155–56, 159–61, 164–65, 173, 183, 190–91
  second trimester after birth 173–79
  third trimester after birth 181–87
  two-a-day program 191
  type 112–23
EXERCISE TRACKERS
  during pregnancy 144
  first six weeks 160–61
  how to use 154–55
  one-a-day program 191
  second trimester after birth 174–79
  third trimester after birth 183
  weeks six to 12 165
EXERCISES
  abdominal 157–59, 186
    crunches 167–68
  arm crossover 163
  back extension 168–69, 177
  back stretch 149
  biceps curl 193
  cat stretch 148
  chest
    fly 194–95
    opener 149, 162, 170
  crossover back stretch 178
  crunches on ball 196
  dumbbell row 195
  hip rotation 147
  inner-thigh stretch 150
  leg curl 192–93
  lower back stretch 163
  lunges 176
    dynamic 184
    travelling 184
  neck stretch 151, 163
  oblique crunch 176
  pelvic floor muscle 145, 156–57
  plank 175
  push-ups 146–47, 175
    on toes 185
    princess 166
    wall 166
  seated toe touch 151, 163
  shoulder roll 162
  stamina 162, 166, 183
  strength 162, 166, 175, 184
  stretching 162, 169, 178, 186, 196
  squats 145, 168, 185
  thigh stretch 150
  triceps
    and shoulder stretch 148, 170, 185
    extension 193
    dip 177–78
  upright row 194

fat 55–57
  low- 100, 102
  recommended intake 69
fitness
  definition 109–11
  goals 134–35
F.I.T.T formula 114
food diary 14, 85–88
  labels 79
food pyramid 67–68
  for breastfeeding mums 74–75

glycaemic index 60
golden rules for eating 75–76
gym
  equipment at home 130–34
  equipment wish list 134
  pros and cons of joining 129–30

habits, kicking bad 13–18

interval training 121

junk food 78

Karvonen formula 118
kilocalories (Kcal) 48–49
kilojoules (kJ) 47, 48–49
K.I.S.S. philosophy, definition 20

lifestyle pyramid 68

meal inspiration 93–100
metabolism 45
  definition 46–47, 49
  basal metabolic rate, definition 47
  during pregnancy and breastfeeding 47–48
  resting metabolic rate, definition 47
  set point theory 47
muscle strength 111–13

pantry staples 88, 90–91
pelvic floor muscle
  identifying 156
  exercise 145, 156–57
perceived exertion 118–19
Plan B, definition, 4
planning, how to 33–42
  meals 35–36
portion control 80–82
postnatal depression, see baby blues
protein 61
  recommended intake 69

repetitions, see sets and repetitions
resistance training 111–13
resting metabolic rate, definition 47

saturated fat 55
set point theory 47
sets and repetitions, definition 155
shopping for food 92–93
stress, definition 21
Supermum syndrome 22–24

TABLES
  3.1 my schedule 40
  4.1 BMI classification 50
  5.1 kJ/day for healthy weight 69
  5.2 junk food/better choices 78
  7.1 rate of perceived exertion 118
  8.1 pregnancy exercise tracker 144
  8.2 example pregnancy exercise tracker 144
  9.1 first six weeks 160
  9.2 example first six weeks 161
  9.3 weeks six to 12 165
  10.1 second trimester after birth 174
  11.1 third trimester after birth 183
  12.1 one-a-day program 191
  12.2 two-a-day program 191
target heart rate 115–19
time-saving strategies 35–39
trans fats 56

unsaturated fat 55–56

vitamins 69–70

water 70–72, 74
weight supported/bearing exercise 123–27
workout examples 120